Hey Cancer, F**K You!

A Memoir with a Message

Lewis Shaw, MD

ISBN: 9781095267912
ISBN-13: 9781095267912

Cover Photo: Molly Diodato

Because of Pat Shaw

HEY CANCER, F**K YOU!

CONTENTS

Prologue	Pg.1
Incidentally	Pg. 4
A Diagnosis	Pg. 6
“The Weight”	Pg. 10
The Pretreatment Interlude	Pg. 17
A View from the Bed	Pg. 21
Cliché Alert	Pg. 26
An Epiphany	Pg. 29
Scramblin Man	Pg. 31
A Dolphin Laughs at Me – The Odyssey Continues	Pg. 34
“Mellow Yellow”	Pg. 37
This is Ridicoulous – Strike One	Pg. 39
“Green Grass and High Tides	Pg. 46
Cosmic Bad Luck	Pg. 48
The Unexpected	Pg. 50
“Keep Pushin”	Pg. 55
An Unexpected Question	Pg. 58
Not That Brave and Not Very Smart	Pg. 59
Cosmic Good Luck	Pg. 61
This is Ridiculous – Strike Two	Pg. 63

"My Silver Lining" Pg. 66

I Won't Do That Again Pg. 69

"Simple Man" Pg. 73

A Moment In Time Pg. 75

This is Ridiculous – Strike Three Pg. 76

Behind Yellow Eyes Pg. 80

"Darkness, Darkness" Pg. 82

A Moment of Transcendence Pg. 84

Bumps in the Road Pg. 87

"Strength" Pg. 93

A Tea Party Pg. 99

Asking an Unexpected Question Pg. 101

Ten Years After Pg. 102

Decision-Making and Integrating Treatment Pg. 105

That which is True Pg. 109

Appendices Pg. 112

PROLOGUE

There is nothing good about having incurable cancer, NOTHING!

It should not take a diagnosis of incurable cancer to make you appreciate life and its blessings. When diagnosed with a serious form of an incurable disease you will view your life from a new perspective. Having no correctable regrets about your life and being at peace with your faith become stunningly important.

What follows is the factual account of my odyssey as a cancer patient, all of it true. I'm an Emergency Physician. Prior to being diagnosed with cancer, at some point every day, I realized how fortunate I was not being a patient and at some point after every shift I ever worked, I hoped that when I became a patient I would cope with grace and some humor.

Nothing can fully prepare you for the patient experience, even being a doctor. For me, more than the suffering, the experience has been about wasted time. Other than giving birth to a healthy baby, being a patient is an enormous waste of time. There are hundreds of things a normal person would rather do with their time than be a patient.

The following will help explain the story telling aids I use in this book:

Some of the chapter titles are song titles. The song or a passage of the song is particularly pertinent to the events in the chapter. Admiration, great appreciation and thanks to the musical artists as the named songs and many others by many other artists are part of my ongoing music therapy.

Frequently I talk to and with myself. Sometimes aloud in order to determine how it sounds when I speak a thought or to practice portions of anticipated conversations. Often the remark or conversation is silent, clear and distinct but silent. Words, phrases, sentences and discussions contained within the < and > signs are an accurate narrative of what my mind was saying at that moment in time. For example a discussion with myself might proceed as follows:

Many people think it's a sign of mental illness if one talks with oneself… A popular misconception. It's only a sign of mental illness if one truly believes or perceives that two separate and distinct individuals are conversing… You hope… No, I'm sure.

These conversations have many benefits such as the healthy expression of anger, frustration, joy, etc. when vocal expression is inappropriate… True and I get the opportunity to discuss an issue or formulate an argument against someone who is objective and who does not have a conflict of interest.>

The reader gets the idea.

Cliché alert warns the reader that a cliché immediately follows. A cliché is an expression of an idea that has been overused to the point of being worn out. At one time the cliché was effective, but it has been repeated so many times it has lost its original impact. Although by definition unoriginal, there is almost universal understanding of a cliché in its culture of origin. With apologies in advance, I occasionally use clichés because of the instant, widespread understanding.

Brackets, [ ] enclose a statement directed toward a specific individual or individuals, such as [Thank you for spending time to read this.]

I am challenged by nonfunctioning pancreatic neuroendocrine cancer, a rare disease. A huge challenge for patients having a rare disease with multiple therapeutic options is that typically there are seldom good comparative effectiveness trials to help us decide which treatment is best because not enough matched patients can be enrolled in each treatment group to reach statistically valid conclusions. Additionally, expert opinion is partially determined by the bias of the expert and such biases might persist for some time after evidence for alternate treatment becomes available. Finally, true experts in rare diseases are few and far between. Thus the circumstances of having a rare disease helped create my odyssey.

Special thanks to my cousin Judy Stockey and my friend Betsy Hancock for encouraging me to write this book.

Profound thanks to friends Rena Fox for editing the manuscript and Steve Barnhart for his critique.

And so it began…

INCIDENTALLY

I was daydreaming when it started. It was about 6 p.m. and the February 24, 2004 meeting of the PinnacleHealth System's Medical Executive Committee was well underway. However, as the topic under discussion did not involve my department or anyone in it, I was thinking about the upcoming weekend when I felt a twinge. Truly that's all it was. A twinge just below my ribs on the right side in the front. The remainder of the meeting and evening passed uneventfully.

When I woke the next morning I was different. My body had changed overnight. My life was about to change forever. My lifelong skinny, flat abdomen was distended, significantly distended in the upper right quarter.

The associated feeling of painful pressure extended to the right side of my mid- back. Finally on the surface of my abdomen there was a visibly distended vein coursing between my umbilicus (bellybutton) and the bottom of my breastbone. I walked downstairs to the kitchen and showed my wife, Stephanie.

"What's that?" she asked.

"I don't know." was my brilliant response. Briefly I tried to think of a clever quip about pregnancy because earlier that month Stephanie told me it was time to start planning for our second child. I was unsuccessful. My mind was preoccupied. I didn't know what was happening. Instead I just said, "I need to go to the ED (Emergency Department) and get this evaluated."

As I drove to the hospital I was thinking how to dovetail being evaluated as a patient with my workday. I had finished thinking about diagnostic possibilities by the time I exited the driveway. I didn't know what this was and I needed a CAT[1] scan.

My colleague and friend, Lance, was on duty and consequently he became the first physician to join me on my odyssey. He ordered an ultrasound, so off to Imaging I went. The ultrasound tech's face told me that something was amiss, but I already knew that.

As I trusted her for a good preliminary report, I asked. She correctly replied that she was not permitted to give a patient her interpretation of the study. She summoned the radiologist who performed some scanning of her own and reviewed the images with me.

My signs and symptoms were being caused by a cyst into which there had been extensive bleeding. She confirmed the need for CAT scan. I went back to the ED, then subsequently to the CAT scanner. The radiologist reviewed the CAT scan images with me. Indeed I had a liver cyst, probably congenital or developmental which had expanded to about 7 inches in size because of bleeding. The cyst was compressing my right kidney causing back pain, the radiologist explained.

"Incidentally the rest of your liver isn't normal," he continued.

---

[1] CAT scan – Computerized Axial Tomography scan. A diagnostic radiological imaging technique in which ionizing radiation is used to obtain an image of a single cross-sectional plane by computer synthesis of the x-ray data from different directions in the given plane. Its development and 1970s revolutionized medical diagnostic imaging.

A DIAGNOSIS

"What do you mean 'isn't normal'? " I asked.

"There are multiple abnormal areas in your liver including one about 8 cm (3 inches) in size, which should be easy to biopsy," replied the radiologist.

<I need a biopsy. That's not good.>

"Okay, when can the biopsy be performed?" was my next question.

"That will probably depend on your disposition, whether you're admitted or not."

The remainder of Wednesday morning was unique. It's not good to be an interesting patient in your own department, or in anyone's department for that matter, because interesting means an uncommon and/or unfortunate diagnosis or situation. I was evaluated by gastroenterology, general surgery and transplant surgery and everyone was playing the "Guess What the Biopsy Will Show" game.

The decision was made to admit me to the hospital for observation in case the cyst ruptured and to expedite the MRI[2] and the biopsy. I'd never answered so many questions about myself as I did that Wednesday. Question after question about the present situation, my past medical history, past surgical history, social history and family history. As I heard myself answer the questions, repeating many of the answers for each specialty service, I became more perplexed. What the heck could this be? In between evaluations I was busy socializing. There was a steady stream of well-wishers and curiosity seekers.

---

[2] MRI – Magnetic Resonance Imaging. A diagnostic radiological imaging technique in which a strong, uniform magnetic field is to obtain images. Unlike conventional diagnostic radiographic imaging or computerized axial tomographic (CAT) scanning, MRI does not expose the patient to ionizing radiation.

Day 2 of my odyssey began with a MRI. The MRI was interesting. Wrapped snugly I slid into the gantry. The gantry made for a tight cocoon, but it was not uncomfortable. The inside of the gantry was white and about 3 to 4 inches from my eyes. The blue line indicating the midline of the gantry was the only non-white thing in my field of vision, but because it was so close I got cross eyed when I looked at it. With closed eyes required, my attention focused on sound and touch.

Although moderately loud the chugging machine-like noise of the scanner was ultimately white noise. Touch focused on the cool breeze flowing past my face.

<This isn't bad. I might be able to take a nap, but it's the wrong time of day and I'm listening to music.>

My thoughts drifted to a conversation with my dad from several years earlier. He had been admitted to a hospital for evaluation of vertigo and had just returned to his room from having a MRI of his head. I had never seen him agitated, but he was very agitated then.

"I'll never have one of those again!" he pronounced.

"Okay dad, no one is saying that you need to have another one," I replied, trying to talk him down.

"I don't care what it means, I will not go through that again."

"Okay dad, okay. No one will force you to have another one. Did something happen?" I continued.

"No, nothing happened," he asserted. "Never again."

Very curious, I thought, but given his level of agitation at the time I wasn't going to resurrect that topic. I would simply have to remain curious.

Left alone Wednesday evening I was able to go downstairs to my office and get some work done. As no one could do my work for me, getting work done in the times in between became essential.

On Thursday there was a very small audience for my biopsy. Lance, my friend and longtime colleague asked the radiologist performing the biopsy if he could tell from the feel of the needle entering the tissue what type of lesion it was. He could not. The remainder of Thursday passed uneventfully. More visits with family, friends, colleagues and coworkers and rounds by the various physicians.

While waiting for the results of an important test physicians can't resist speculating about the results, it's our nature. The speculation voiced by my treating physicians focused on fibronodular or focal nodular hyperplasia of the liver as my diagnosis. I was informed that I was to be discharged the next day. The quiet of the hospital evening arrived and I returned to my office to work.

Friday morning, family present, I was dressed and waiting for physician rounds and completion of the discharge process. Summarizing my status and treatment plan the transplant surgeon said that an outpatient appointment to have the cyst drained would be scheduled and the biopsy results would be available Monday providing the definitive diagnosis.

"Sometimes we see what we want to see," he said, "but it appears you have fibronodular hyperplasia. So while we will be ready in the bullpen, your liver is sustaining you for now and you don't need us. You will follow up with Steve (gastroenterologist)."

<I know almost nothing about fibronodular hyperplasia. I know what I'll be reading about this weekend.>

Family members said their goodbyes and left. I was discharged and returned to my office to work. Workday complete I was anxious to get home. Walking to the parking garage I saw my gastroenterologist, Steve headed toward the hospital.

"Hi Steve," I said.

"We need to talk," He replied.

As you know nothing good ever follows that line and I felt doom. We entered the hospital via a side door and walked into the administrative suite. Steve found an open, empty office and we sat down.

"You have a tumor." He said

"THE WEIGHT"
The Band
February 27 – March 3, 2004

"Jules P. (PinnacleHealth pathologist) called me," Steve said. "He read your slides and favors primary hepatocellular (liver cell) cancer."

<Nothing>

"Although he says it could be metastatic renal (kidney) cancer or carcinoid. They sent slides to the Fox Chase Cancer Center (FCCC) for special staining to make a definitive diagnosis. They said we should have the results Monday."

<Nothing>

"Do you have any siblings?" Steve continued.

"One sister," I replied, proving capable of speech.

"Is she in good health?"

"Yes."

"If it proves to be hepatocellular cancer, the recommend treatment will be a living donor liver transplant and it will need to be performed as soon as it can be arranged. You should talk with your sister," Steve concluded.

"Okay."

"Who do you want as your oncologist?" Steve asked.

"Ron Alexander, if he's taking new patients," I replied instantly. Having observed Dr. Roland (Ron) Alexander professionally for more than 15 years I knew him to be thoughtfully intelligent, diligent, compassionate and always have the moral high ground. I had most closely observed these and many other positive qualities during the years he cared for one of my Emergency Physician colleagues during her war with breast cancer.

"I'll talk with Ron and I'm sure he'll contact you to follow up. I'm sorry."

"Thanks Steve, me too."

As we exited the office we happened upon one of the vice presidents who offered his sincere condolences and any help he could provide.

<Bad news travels fast.>

After thanking the vice president, Steve and I parted ways. Again I was heading home, but my agenda had been slightly altered. Instead of a restful weekend spent reading about fibronodular hyperplasia, I needed to tell my loved ones I had a menacing cancer and ask my sister for part of her liver. A massive, oppressive, unimaginable obligation I thought as I walked to the parking garage.

As I drove out of the parking garage I considered how I would accomplish these tasks. My mind flicked through potential scenarios because each and every one was too heavy to contemplate. Worse, there was no script. Worse yet, traffic was moving very well for Friday evening rush hour and I was getting to my destination much too quickly.

<How am I going to do this? This is suffocating. This is intolerable.>

At that very moment the "check engine" light flashed on my dashboard. The cosmic theater-of-the- absurd was reminding me that…

cliché alert

…life goes on, and as my sense of humor tends to lie in the absurd, I chuckled.

<Just tell everyone, ask your sister and push on.>

The only thing I remember and have ever remembered about telling Stephanie was the back drop, our happy three year old son, Nate; too young to understand and too young to remember his father if I was to die in the near future.

I drove to my sister's house and, as her family was also at home, I asked her to walk with me for a few minutes. I briefly explained the situation and asked her for part of her liver.

While it was the most difficult question I've ever asked, in the instant I asked it I knew it was the easiest to answer. Also in that instant I began to hate this disease with an absolute, profoundness which startled me. I hadn't known I was capable of pure hate.

Surprisingly, telling my parents was not difficult, but experiencing their reaction was. For their generation cancer was a death sentence. In their eyes I could see abject horror at the prospect of burying their only son. I'm not sure if it was because my dad's mind fused at that point, but Mom was first to comprehend their only daughter as a liver donor.

<Yes Mom it can always get worse.>

The next day was very challenging because the news was so overwhelming I couldn't think beyond getting a definitive diagnosis and implication of each of the three possible diagnoses. I certainly was not capable of being productive. My dad's mind wasn't the only one stuck. A day hike was suggested and it seemed like an excellent idea.

So the next day, Sunday was spent hiking on the Appalachian Trail with family (figure 1). It was good to move, get some fresh air and spend time with family. I began to get my mind unstuck. First the differential diagnosis. Every patient I had ever seen with metastatic kidney cancer felt and looked sick, so unlikely to be that.

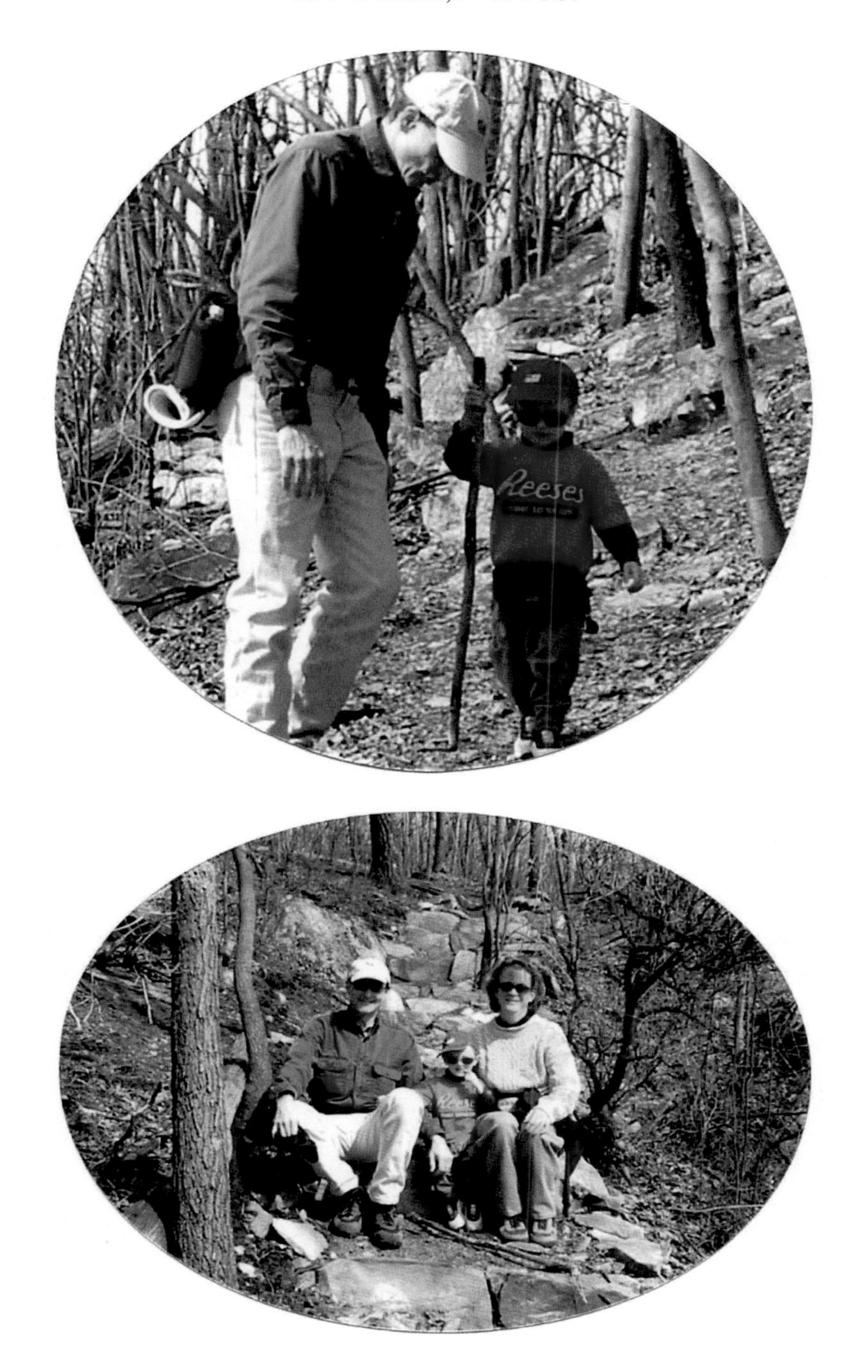

Figure 1 – Getting my mind unstruck on the Appalachian Trail. February 29, 2004

Every patient I had ever seen with multiple lesions of primary liver cell cancer felt sick and was yellow, so again, unlikely. Consequently I concluded metastatic carcinoid cancer was most likely; but what if my experience as a non-oncologist, non-gastroenterologist was misleading. I would just have to wait.

Much more important was establishing goals. Always having goals is fundamental to a good life. The first goal was easy to establish, outlive my parents; because no parent should have to bury their child. As I walked and interacted with my son the second goal came to mind. As I'd taken on the earthly responsibility of a child, I needed to get him to the age of majority, only 15 years to go. The final goal was each and every day to be better than I was the day before. It was a good hike.

Monday was typical at work except for the undercurrent of anticipation of a tissue diagnosis. However, there was no diagnosis that day or the next. By the end of Tuesday I was about out of adjectives to describe the wait; unbearable, oppressive, unmanageable, intolerable, insufferable, egregious. Yep, that about covered it. Every time I shuffled and dealt the diagnostic possibilities I came up with carcinoid, but maybe that was only wishful thinking as carcinoid cancer was least likely to kill me quickly. On my way to work Wednesday I deposited my vehicle at the service garage to have that "check engine" light evaluated. When I retrieved it after work, I had a diagnosis for the vehicle but not for myself.

At least I won't fret away this evening I thought as I was driving home. My friend Logan was visiting from California and would be at my house. As we sat chatting the phone rang.

I answered it. "Hello?"

"Hi Lew, it's Ron Alexander."

"Hi Ron."

"How are you doing?"

<How am I doing?! HOW AM I DOING?! I'll tell you how I'm doing. I'm about ready to "blow an O-ring[3]" waiting for this diagnosis. That's

[3] This refers to the catastrophic mechanical failure which resulted in the spectacular

how I'm doing. Give me the diagnosis already!>

Dr. Alexander was starting to train me as a patient. Of course there was a result, but at least as important as the result was 'How are you, the patient doing?' Over the years he would impress upon me how patients and physicians can obsess about a test result to the detriment of the patient; by losing sight of the foundation of the situation, what is the patient's overall status, 'How are you doing?'

"Except for the distention from the cyst, I feel fine," I tried to say calmly.

"Good. The FCCC pathologist says it's a neuroendocrine cancer."

"Is that related to carcinoid cancer?"

"Not bad for an ER doc. It will give you something to read about before you see me in the office. Do you need anything?"

"Other than a cure, no."

"Call me if you need anything."

"Okay. Thanks, bye."

"Goodbye."

"Well?" Stephanie asked anxiously.

"He says it's neuroendocrine cancer," I replied.

"What's that?" she asked.

"It's related to carcinoid cancer and it's a rare. Otherwise I don't know much about it."

"So it's the best of the three possibilities?"

"Seems to be. At least no immediate liver transplant."

---

destruction of the space shuttle Challenger shortly after takeoff in January, 1986.

The wait for a diagnosis had been interminable. What I didn't know at the time was that, as much as anything else, this odyssey would be about waiting. Scheduling appointments, studies and lab tests. Preparing and travelling for the appointments, studies and tests. The appointments, studies and tests themselves. Waiting at every step. All an enormous waste of time as there are always innumerable things I would rather be doing than dealing with this disease.

THE PRETREATMENT INTERLUDE

The next two weeks were chaotic.

I was still adjusting to my role as Chair of Emergency Medicine, having started that job three months prior to diagnosis. Not only was this disease not helping my professional adjustment, but also I had to adjust to having a bad disease about which I knew precious little. The external pressure to perform superbly as Chair was intense. The internal pressure to start treatment was intense. Best not to let either intrude on the other. Work was work, no distractions. The disease immediately became an extracurricular activity, my hobby. Reading, studying, thinking every evening after my three-year-old son went to bed, hoping not to get distracted by a phone call or a page from work.

Shortly after becoming Chair I realized the more I talked the longer my work days were. Additionally I learned more by listening and then I did by talking. Consequently I attempted to keep my part of professional conversations to a minimum. At work I extended this conversation guideline to the topic of my disease. The nature of fast traveling bad news made it obvious I shouldn't spend any precious time or effort attempting to hide my disease; so I engaged any conversation initiated about my disease being open, honest and brief for my part. To some of the people at work I was already gone. It is a very peculiar look some people give those who they believe to have a terminal disease when the incurable ones are not a family member or a close friend. Receiving those looks in passing at the hospital or at meetings probably would have been more disquieting if I had completely processed the circumstances. As it was, I was mostly curious about the looks because I hadn't undergone one day of treatment.

Within 48 hours of receiving the diagnosis I met with my accountant. The meeting was a previously scheduled, routine annual tax preparation appointment. My accountant was a very smart dude with an outstanding sense of how the world works. He had earned my respect. Consequently he grabbed my total attention when without hesitation he told me to complete the required paperwork and "go out on disability" in order to devote all of my time and effort to fighting the cancer. Our meeting ended and I walked out of his office considering his recommendation about disability, firmly rejecting it before I got to my car.

Dovetailing work with that initial evaluation as a patient was the first, simplest step of a long formidable journey. There were more consultations, evaluations and pretreatment planning to squeeze into the two weeks before my first treatment and, lest you've forgotten, there was a cyst to be drained. Although I was no longer worried that the cyst would spontaneously rupture resulting in who knew how much bleeding into my abdomen, I was concerned any minor injury would cause the same result. Its size restricted movement of my torso, my ability to breathe deeply and therefore my ability to exercise. The pain was annoying and I didn't like the fact that one of my kidneys was being compressed. Each day something accreted. An endocrinology consult, additional preparation for the first treatment, cyst drainage, a routine dental exam and cleaning prior to chemo and its attendant immunocompromise.

Finally I was in Dr. Ron Alexander's office for an initial evaluation and I felt fortunate to be there because of my high regard for him, professionally and personally.

"Blah, blah, blah," I heard as he began his introductory remarks which seemed scripted. His script would have been carefully crafted during the decades of seeing newly diagnosed cancer patients.

"Blah, blah…PALLIATIVE CARE," he continued.

<PALLIATIVE CARE! What the what, that means I'm dying!!>

He must have known the term 'palliative care' would command my attention and begin the process of accepting my disease as incurable. I heard his every word the remainder of the appointment.

"I discussed your case with Dr. E. at the Fox Chase Cancer Center and we agree the first step is to direct treatment at the large liver lesion by embolizing[4] it. While he agrees there is no good evidence that adding cytotoxic drugs to the embolization process adds anything but toxicity, chemoembolization is typically what they do there." Ron continued, "At University of Pittsburgh Medical Center (UPMC) they also typically perform their liver embolizations with chemo. Although Pittsburgh is not as convenient as Philadelphia for you, I prefer you go there for your chemoembolization."

"Why?" I asked.

"You'll be treated at their Liver Cancer Center with its attendant transplant program. That way if you end up needing a liver transplant because of treatment complications, they will already own you."

"Understood. I have extended family in Pittsburgh so I'll feel a lot better having them nearby."

"Good, we'll make the arrangements."

I received many phone calls during those two weeks. As you would expect most were kind inquiries, condolences and/or sincere offers to help. One call was very different. The call was from my cousin Mira, a very experienced nurse in a transplant program in Arizona. We chatted for a while. I described the situation and told her the agreed-upon first treatment was hepatic chemo embolization. She said the treatment would make me feel "puny." Then she said if treatment came to a liver transplant that I could have part of her liver, assuming it was an appropriate match. Stunned, I started to mumble a response, but she cut me off. She said she had already talked to her husband and gotten medical leave of absence approval from her supervisor. In the way of a disclaimer she mentioned her liver might not be in perfect shape as it had endured some partying when she was younger, "as you know," but I was still welcome to part of it. "Heroic" was the single word which instantly came to mind and with respect to cousin Mira it has never left.

---

[4] The therapeutic introduction of a substance to occlude the blood flow of a vessel such that blood no longer flows beyond the obstructing embolus. In this situation to devitalize the tumor resulting in its death (necrosis).

Stephanie and I always planned to have more than one child and, as previously mentioned, in early February she informed me it was time to try for our second child. Although she had not mentioned the topic since my diagnosis, generic items from our son's infancy, kept for our next child, began to appear in the garbage and in the pile for charity.

A VIEW FROM THE BED

There are only four truly unidirectional, life-will-never-be-the-same events: the first time one falls in love, exiting school/training to enter the adult workforce/military service, becoming a parent and the transition from good health to a state of chronic disease. Being a physician did not prepare me for the loss of my good health or for being a patient with an incurable disease.

The first stop on my odyssey as a patient was the UPMC's Liver Cancer Center for hepatic artery chemoembolization treatment (HACE)[5]. The experience was my first exposure to protocol medicine as a patient and my first opportunity to be a good patient. The treatments were rigidly choreographed; arrive on Monday for clinic visit, lab studies and CT scanning, return early Tuesday morning for HACE treatment followed by admission to the hospital, discharge to home Wednesday after laboratory and physician evaluation. My first treatment in March, 2004 was a real eye-opener.

On Monday everything happened smoothly and as anticipated. The oncologist (Dr. C.) was very direct and spoke assertively.

"We must control the liver," he said. "Give me 4 to 6 months to make sure the liver is controlled and we'll discuss the next steps and overall plan." That sounded very reasonable to my wife and me.

Early Tuesday morning I arrived at the pre-procedure area to be prepped for the HACE treatment. Part of the preparation was placement of a Foley catheter through my penis into my bladder to drain urine. Because I knew Foley catheter insertion to be a painful procedure, I requested a small catheter and that an anesthetic lubricant be instilled prior to catheter insertion. I was informed that neither a small catheter nor anesthetic lubricant were readily available and that things needed to

[5] In Hepatic Artery Chemoembolization (HACE) treatment a catheter is inserted into the femoral artery in the groin. The catheter is then advanced/threaded up through the hepatic (liver) artery into the artery supplying blood to the tumor. A chemotherapy drug is given through the catheter directly into the tumor. The artery is then embolized to block the blood flow to the tumor.

"move along". Sometimes the anticipation of an event is worse than the event itself, not in this instance. It hurt, a lot. The bright red blood draining into the urine collection bag reassured me that I wasn't being excessively wimpy. Shortly after the worst part of the preparation came the best, lorazepam (Ativan) given intravenously to reduce anxiety. After signing consent for the procedure I was given intravenous lorazepam.

<This is delightful! Now I understand why some people abuse Ativan.>

Since I hadn't felt anxious about the HACE procedure itself, the lorazepam moved me directly to a happy, chatty, less inhibited state of mind. It was the only pleasant aspect of the entire ordeal. After the HACE treatment I felt very puny for about 4 days and full recovery from the procedure required about 4 weeks. Mira's one word summary was accurate.

Recovery from the first treatment was punctuated by my three-year-old son's first joke, at my expense of course. As I was losing heaps of hair, I stopped on my way home from work one day to have my remaining hair shaved off. Arriving home my wife and son waited at the door to greet me. On exiting the vehicle my son said,

"Dad, dad what's on your head?"

I reflexively brushed my scalp with my hand to remove any wayward insect or debris.

"What?" I responded not feeling anything foreign on my head.

"Nothing!" he exclaimed laughing.

"Good one," I chuckled.

I was better prepared for my second HACE treatment. I arrived in the preprocedure prep area on Tuesday with my own small Foley catheter and anesthetic lubricant. Although it engendered a few incompletely concealed snickers from the staff, catheter insertion was painless and there was no bleeding. Next came my second misstep as a patient, the first was not insisting on anesthetic lubricant and a small Foley catheter during my first treatment. Some background is needed to set the stage. As a high school student I worked part-time as a phlebotomist at our local medical center. From that perspective it was striking and memorable how patients benefited from having multiple, easily accessible veins. This was especially true for chemotherapy patients as repeated chemotherapy treatments damaged veins making them inaccessible. The patients with good veins experienced much faster, less painful phlebotomy and intravenous (IV) cannula insertions. Medical school and residency reinforced my initial experience and by the end of my training I was a strong advocate of good vein stewardship. Consequently I was paying attention when the nurse missed a very good left forearm vein attempting to insert an IV cannula. She was pleasant, confident and apologized for the miss. Anyone can miss a good vein on occasion, I thought not yet concerned about the procedure. She chatted about her daughter's cell phone bill as she prepared for her next attempt.

<Whoa! Is she really going to attempt the same vein 3 inches farther down the forearm?! She should try a different vein or farther up the forearm if she's going to try the same vein... You should say something... Nah, no way she's going to miss that vein again.>

She missed that vein again, still apparently more concerned about her daughter's cell phone bill than successful IV cannula insertion. Subsequently the 3 inch segment of that vein between the two missed attempts thrombosed (clotted) and became permanently inaccessible. The remainder of the second treatment and recovery occurred as expected.

Karma[6] visited the preprocedure area during my third HACE treatment (June, 2004). All had gone smoothly for me and I was in the Ativan induced happy, chatty, less inhibited state of mind. On the other side of the privacy curtain to my right was a patient being prepped for his first HACE treatment. Additionally I overheard the patient say he had prior intravenous chemotherapy at a different facility.

"After the chemo is injected into the tumor through the catheter in your liver, they inject material to stop the blood flow to the tumor. This helps kill the tumor cells and keeps the chemo from flowing out of the liver, so you won't get sick," explained the same nurse who squandered 3 inches of a great vein during my previous treatment.

[6] Here the term karma is used to denote the concept of fate as a result of cause and effect. The principle being that a person is rewarded or punished at a future time for a deed or action.

“That’s not true,” I said to the curtain. “The chemo eventually exits the liver into your system. I got sick after each of my previous two treatments. I don’t know if you’ll get as sick as you did with the intravenous chemo, but you’ll get sick.”

<Uh oh, you should NOT have said that, she’s not going to like it… Obviously the Ativan is responsible and what I said and it was true and accurate… Still you shouldn’t have said it… Oh well… Yes, oh well>

After the pre-procedure theater my third treatment and post-procedure care proceeded routinely. Wednesday morning Stephanie and my cousin Judy arrived to wait with me for the oncologist to round and write the discharge order. Dr. C. appeared and after examining me reviewed the procedure and labs with us. Everything was as expected. Before leaving the room to write the discharge order and instructions he described a change in routine for the next visit. I was to schedule an early Monday morning CT scan followed by a morning clinic appointment, so we could discuss the overall plan. The requested change would increase the complexity of our travel logistics, but we were glad to oblige. My loved ones and I were eager to learn the recommended overall treatment plan.

August 2004 and time for my fourth HACE treatment. With a Monday morning CT scan and breakfast in the rearview mirror Stephanie and I waited expectantly in the exam room.

“What are you doing here?” Dr. C. pointedly asked as he entered the room.

“You told us to make a morning clinic appointment so we could discuss the overall treatment plan,” I replied.

“Why would I do that? Your CT scan hasn’t been read by radiology. There’s nothing to discuss yet.”
Although speechless I sensed my wife’s dismay and consternation at his comment. “The secretary said you insisted on being seen this morning,” he pressed on.

“We simply did what you told us to do at the time of discharge from my last treatment,” I stated firmly locking his eyes with my gaze.

My wife nodded in agreement. He paused.

"Hung by my own words," he conceded.

With there being nothing to discuss at that time, the clinic visit, HACE treatment and post-procedure recovery went smoothly. At discharge I was instructed to follow the schedule of the first three treatments for my next treatment.

After returning home and getting back to work, I dutifully scheduled my fifth HACE treatment and followed up with Dr. Alexander.

"CLICHÉ ALERT"
FROM THE SUBMLIME TO THE RIDICULOUS
OCTOBER 7, 2004

Our National Cancer Institute (NCI) in Bethesda, Maryland is an amazing place.

While waiting for my fifth HACE treatment Dr. Alexander referred me to the NCI seeking a research study for which I qualified. Ron had impressed upon me the potential benefits of participating in a good experimental study. Having a rare disease means fewer validated treatment options, less consensus on standard therapy, and typically a lack of comparative effectiveness studies[7]. He also impressed upon me the need to have contingency plans A and B ready for when current treatment becomes ineffective. So it was off to the NCI, after the necessary but tedious "new patient dance."

The "new patient dance" is the process in which a patient requests evaluation and/or treatment by a new provider or facility, the new dance partner. The patient must provide the prospective partner with completed questionnaires, scans, lab results, pathology slides, operative notes, admission summaries, insurance information, etc. before the prospective partner will consider accepting the invitation. This process typically takes days to weeks to complete.

On the road at 5 a.m. for an 8 a.m. starting time, it had the potential to be a long day. The worst part of the day, the fast and absence of caffeine would be over by noon. There were no travel or parking problems. Registration, labs and ECG all very efficient. Excellent so far I thought as I walked toward the CAT scan area.

The CAT scan sub-waiting room was almost empty when I arrived. In health care a sub-waiting room is an accessory waiting room designed to

[7] Comparative effectiveness studies are those in which treatment A is compared to treatment B in similar patients to determine which treatment is better. Conducting a comparative effectiveness study for the treatment of a rare disease is very challenging because it is difficult to find enough patients to reach statistically valid conclusions.

cohort (group) patients who are at the same stage of a process. When used for patients who are waiting test results and/or discharge it can make available valuable treatment space for other patients. When used as another location to wait for a test to be performed, it's just that, another place to wait for a test to be performed; but it is one that emphasizes the appearance of progress. The only noteworthy aspect of this sub-waiting room was the evidence of nearby renovations, signs and construction barriers across the hall.

The wait began routinely. I chugged the oral contrast in order to minimize the length time I tasted it. I expected to be in the scanner in an hour. Patients began to trickle in, among them a student, high school judging by her study materials. About an hour into my wait I noticed no one was leaving the sub- waiting room for their scan. A short while later it was announced that our wait time was due to one of the scanners being used for critically ill patients in the ICU. The announcement was accompanied by sincere apologies for our wait.

As the sub-waiting room became crowded the grumbling began. I took a break from my reading and allowed my thoughts to wander. How horrible it must be for this high school student. On the verge of young adulthood and what should be a great time in her life, yet she was in these horrible circumstances. Outwardly she was very calm. To look at her one would think she was in a high school library working on an assignment. The next announcement brought louder grumbling and a few groans, a second scanner was unavailable to us because it was being repaired. Our wait times would be longer. Sincere apologies were again offered and our forbearance was requested. The sub-waiting room was now standing room only and some patients were getting restless, standing in the doorway or walking in the hallway to stretch their legs. They were soon herded back into the sub-waiting room. We were asked not to loiter in the hallway because of the construction. Despite the rising, palpable level of tension in the room, the student remained serene.

Cliché alert

Then came the last straw. It was announced there had been a chemotherapy spill in the third scanner. A hazmat team had been summoned, but the scanner would be out of service until they arrived and cleaned up the spill.

<Wait for it>

"You're telling us," said one of the men testily, "that you spilled some of the stuff you pump into our bodies and we're waiting for a hazmat team to clean it up. Give me a mop and bucket and I'll clean it up. This is ridiculous!"

<There it is>

As these events unfolded over 2+ hours we became increasingly concerned about our individual itineraries. I had missed my MRI time and wondered if they had been notified and when they would fit me in. I suspect all of us were hungry, I certainly was. All of us were definitely cranky, except it seemed for the high school student. It got more surreal a short time later when one of the clerks returned and seeing a few of us in the hallway, politely requested we return to the sub-waiting room because she didn't want to have to call security!

<On a bunch of cancer patients, really?!>

Then she likely prevented a ruckus by telling us we would be moving ahead with our itineraries and returning later in the afternoon for our CAT scans.

"Remember, nothing to eat or drink until you've had your scan," she said as she departed.

AN EPIPHANY
OCTOBER 8, 2004

"You could have had this for 15 years," said Dr. H. of the National Cancer Institute's Tumor Immunology Section, starting to summarize the situation and her recommendations.

The experimental protocol being proposed involved open abdominal surgery during which the blood flow through my liver would be separated and isolated from the remainder of my body. Once isolated my liver would be continuously perfused with melphalan, a cytotoxic chemotherapeutic drug for one hour at an elevated temperature. After the perfusion my liver's plumbing would be reconnected to my systemic circulation. The entire process would take 6-8 hours during which I would be in the operating room with my abdomen open. (I had a momentary Monty Python-esque image of my guts falling out.)

However, because of my existing liver cyst it was possible, once my abdomen was opened and assessed, they would not be able to perform the hepatic perfusion and my abdomen would be closed with no treatment given. While Stephanie did not audibly gasp during Dr. H's description of the procedure, I could sense her unease.

Back on the beltway going home Stephanie and I were chatting.

"I know this disease can be slow-growing and present for years before diagnosis, or be present for years and the patient die of something else, or it's found incidentally at autopsy; but to hear a smart, highly trained physician tell me I might have had this for 15 years is surreal."

"15 years is a long time," Stephanie agreed.

"That would be almost 1/3 of my life, which seems incredible to me."

"She said it can be very slow-growing."

"Very slow-growing… He doesn't have a plan!" I said emphatically.

"What?"

"Remember at our first appointment with Dr. C he said to give him 4 to 6 months to gain control of the liver and he would recommend a plan for overall treatment?"

"Yes."

"Remember our misunderstanding of the last appointment, when we were expecting him to outline an overall treatment plan?"

"Yes."

"It seems to me his plan is to keep ringing the cash register at $42,000 per treatment until my heart can't take anymore doxorubicin (Adriamycin), which will be two more treatments, but he doesn't have an overall treatment plan beyond that. I have systemic disease and I need systemic treatment, I think. There must be a better path."

There on the beltway I quit. As I was driving, Stephanie called UPMC and canceled the upcoming appointment for my fifth HACE treatment.

Through her I informed them I would call if I wanted to reschedule. As became my habit I was depending on Dr. Alexander for guidance.

SCRAMBLIN' MAN
WITH APOLOGIES TO THE ALLMAN BROTHERS BAND

Although all diseases are inconvenient, rare diseases are more so, because, among other features, much greater travel usually is required to obtain an equivalent level of expert care. Frustration grows as we citizens of developed countries are being conditioned to expect everything to be immediately available and, if not, someone is to blame. This dual promise of convenience and ability to assign blame is a deception frequently employed by politicians to hustle votes, but I digress.

While I had adjusted to the reality that my disease is incurable, I had yet to adjust to the absence of a standard, accepted treatment pathway or algorithm. There was a lack of adequately powered research studies[8] to aid in the decision-making. Working full-time and having a family, I wanted the treatment decision-making to be easy. It wasn't and still isn't.

Although I thought quitting UPMC's treatment plan was correct, I had doubts about the NCI protocol. If not the NCI protocol, then what? At the time contingency plans A and B did not exist and I began to feel the all-too-familiar and uncomfortable need to scramble. I knew how to scramble, at least professionally. Every time I arrived to start a shift and there were 10 patients in the waiting room who were already angry at me, I scrambled. Every time there were more patients than beds, I scrambled. Every time multiple ambulances arrived simultaneously, I scrambled. I scrambled almost every shift I ever worked, so how much different could this be? Plus I had Ron.

---

[8] The power of a study is the probability that the study will detect the predetermined treatment effect between two groups, if it exists. If an insufficient number of patients are studied the probability of not detecting a real treatment effect is increased. Other errors in design and enrollment can result in the investigators reporting a treatment effect where there is none. A discussion of research study design, methods, analysis of results and incorporating results into clinical decision-making is far beyond the scope of this book.

We return to action in Dr. Alexander's office on October 12, 2004.

"Did you read their protocol?" asked Dr. Alexander referring to the NCI's hepatic perfusion protocol.

"Yes," I replied.

"Then you know you're not eligible."

"The part about '…for patients with cancers that are only in the liver.'?" I ventured.

"Yes," he confirmed.

"Why did they seemingly offer it to me?"

"Probably because you're a physician and they felt obliged to offer you something. I'm not signing off on it."

"Understood."

"Stopping the treatments in Pittsburgh is probably not a bad idea," he continued.

"What's next?" I asked, feeling the need to scramble well up inside.

"I've talked with Dr. E. at the Fox Chase Cancer Center (FCCC). They have an experimental protocol for which you might be eligible. It's an oral drug in a phase 2 study[9]. We'll make an appointment for you."

"Okay, thanks. Do you have any objections to me seeing a carcinoid/neuroendocrine specialist?"

"Of course not, who do you have in mind?"

"I don't know. Any recommendations?"

---

[9] Phase 2 experimental trials continue to test the safety of the treatment and begin to evaluate how well it will work. Generally they do not compare the treatment under investigation with another treatment or with placebo.

"There are only a few nationally worth seeing and none of my current patients is seeing one of them. You might try Yao at M.D. Anderson."

"Okay."

"Let me know what you decide and we'll make the referral."

"Thanks."

Less than three weeks later I was in Philadelphia at the FCCC being evaluated by Dr. E. He confirmed that I was likely eligible for a phase 2 trial and concurred with Dr. Alexander that it would not be advisable for me to undergo the NCI hepatic perfusion protocol.

Regarding carcinoid/neuroendocrine cancer specialists Dr. Alexander was correct. There were only a handful of such specialists in the U.S.A. and none of them nearby. I followed Dr. Alexander's subtle recommendation regarding Dr. Yao at the M.D. Anderson Cancer Center in Houston Texas, initiated the "new patient dance" and made an appointment to see Dr. Yao.

A DOLPHIN LAUGHS AT ME – THE ODYSSEY CONTINUES

Seeking treatment for chronic disease is a form of shopping, with all of the associated implications. I was going shopping in Houston, Texas.

<WOW!>

That was my impression of the new patient intake process at the M.D. Anderson Cancer Center in Houston, Texas. Although accustomed to simultaneous processing of many people for the same purpose, such as admission to an entertainment venue, this was my first experience with it at a health care facility. Oodles of cancer patients handing off piles of medical records from outside facilities, being registered, photographed for the patient ID band, interviewed and directed for testing. Efficient and by its nature impersonal.

In route to the phlebotomy area by elevator I checked my itinerary. As expected only a chest x-ray and a CAT scan of my abdomen and pelvis after phlebotomy.

<Why do most centers insist on their own up-to-the-minute CAT scan, is it just to ‘ring the register’? What’s this, rectal contrast!? That’s almost certainly not going to provide any useful information. Should I decline? It will be a waste of time to ask about the rectal contrast because the response will be “It’s protocol.” or something similar. I can’t say that I’ve already had it because I haven’t. Well, I have a little time to ruminate about it.>

After having my blood drawn and chest x-ray taken I reported to the CAT scan prep area.

<Given that I’ve never undergone CAT scanning with rectal contrast and I don’t want to be a difficult patient, I won’t decline; but I know it’s not going to provide any useful information. Frustrating!>

Sadly, I was already familiar with the CAT scan prep process from the patient perspective. A large, well lit room with many comfortable patient chairs. The patients, most accompanied by a family member or other support person, were drinking contrast, having IVs inserted and waiting. The staff was friendly, attentive and competent and they attempted to lighten the mood. I was not, however, familiar with rectal contrast from the patient perspective. On rare occasions I had been required to insert the enema catheter for the administration rectal contrast and it never endeared me to a patient. My wait ended and I was about to become familiar with rectal contrast from the patient perspective.

Lying on my side on the hard room temperature CAT scan table the enema catheter was inserted. As the contrast begin to flow I hoped this would provide some useful information. No, just rationalizing my decision I concluded as I became more frustrated. With all of the contrast instilled, the catheter was removed. Shortly thereafter I was instructed to roll onto my back. When I did I looked up and was greeted by a picture on the ceiling. The photo was of a grinning dolphin dancing on its tail backwards on top of the water. This photo perfectly depicted the Dolphin's happy, chattering vocalizations. The caption read: "Take time to giggle."

<Come here Flipper, I've got your "giggle" right here!>

The radiologist's report of this pancreatic protocol CAT scan included the statement "the pancreas is unremarkable." (Figure 1). As we all know my primary tumor is in the pancreas.

My shopping trip to Houston included an evaluation at the Burzynski Clinic.

Although the shopping trip to Houston was very informative, as with my trip to the National Cancer Institute, nothing seemed to fit. Concomitantly I was deemed eligible for inclusion in the phase 2 research study of a new drug at the Fox Chase Cancer Center in Philadelphia. The new year, 2005, would bring new treatment and new challenges.

SHAW, LEWIS

DIAGNOSTIC IMAGING CONSULTATION

PATIENT: **SHAW, LEWIS**
PATIENT CLASS: WMMP
PATIENT TYPE: O
RM#: -
CITY/ST/COUNTRY: HUMMELSTOWN, PA UNITED STATES
LOCATION: 444
REQUESTING M.D.: JAMES C. YAO
ORDER NO: 90002
EXAMINATION: **CT, PELVIS W/CONTRAST, on 12/28/2004**

Examination: CT scan of the abdomen and pelvis with contrast, and abdomen without contrast, pancreatic protocol, 12/28/04.

Clinical History: Patient with low grade neuroendocrine cancer with liver metastases. Patient has had chemoembolization and chemotherapy.

IMPRESSION:

1. Multiple enhancing lesions in both lobes of the liver.
2. Large cystic area in the right lobe of the liver possibly secondary to previous chemo embolization.

FULL RESULT: CT scan of the abdomen and pelvis was performed with oral, rectal and IV contrast. Pancreatic protocol was performed.

The lower lungs are unremarkable.

The liver has metastatic lesions in both lobes of the liver. These are hypervascular. There is no significant intrahepatic biilary dilatation at this moment. There is a large cystic lesion in the right lobe of the liver which measures 9.6 cm across. The portal veins are intact. I have no comparison films at this time.

The spleen is normal. the pancreas is unremarkable. The gallbladder is normal.

There is peripancreatic lymphadenopathy. The largest node is 2.1 cm in diameter and is immediately superior to the head of the pancreas between the bifurcation of the celiac artery. There are small nodes in the peri porta hepatis. There is an enlarged node in the left retroperitoneum at the level of the renal artery. I see no other retroperitoneal, pelvic, or inguinal adenopathy.

Both adrenal glands are normal. Both kidneys are functioning without evidence of hydronephrosis or masses. The bladder is normal. The prostate is unremarkable.

The visualized skeleton is unremarkable.

DATE OF INTERPRETATION: Dec 29 2004 9:17A
TRANS BY: jaj at Dec 29 2004 9:45A
TECHNOLOGIST:
Page: 1 of 2
SHAW/634125
ACCESSION#: 4578779

DIAGNOSTIC RADIOLOGY **CT, PELVIS W/CONTRAST**

figure 1.

"MELLOW YELLOW"
DONOVAN

By March, 2005 I was enrolled in a phase 2 research study of Sutent (sunitinib) in patients with advanced neuroendocrine tumors at the Fox Chase Cancer Center. Phase 2 studies evaluate safety and efficacy of a treatment for a disease or condition. Drugs undergo extensive preclinical testing via in vitro (in an artificial environment such as a test tube) and animal experimentation to select those most likely to work in humans. Pharmaceutical companies test over 1.5 million new compounds annually, of which less than one in 5000 advance to testing in phase 1 trials.

Phase 1 trials seek a safe human dosage, dosing frequency and sometimes route of administration. Phase 1 trials also study side effect profiles. Phase 1 trials typically enroll a small number of patients and are not designed to determine the effectiveness of the treatment. Phase 3 studies typically compare the efficacy of the drug to placebo (an inert substance) or some other treatment and are often pivotal in the approval process and in ushering the drug into routine clinical use, or not. Less than one in five drugs entering phase 1 testing successfully complete phase 3 study. The protocol of this particular study specified a clinic visit at the beginning and end of each drug cycle.

I presented myself for the clinic visit at the end of cycle number one.

"Your description of the rash was perfect," said the oncology fellow. She was referring to a widespread rash I developed shortly after starting Sutent. I called her when the rash first appeared, one to two weeks prior to my appointment. Now she was seeing the rash for the first time.

"I endeavor to be precise," I responded using Mr. Spock's line but not his intonation or inflection. Admittedly my reference was very obscure and I did not expect her to acknowledge it.

"You're also yellow," she added, not acknowledging the reference.

"That started just 2 to 3 days ago. Since I was scheduled to see you it seemed reasonable not to bother you with a call."

"Most patients I've seen get very anxious when they turn yellow and call immediately."

"You did an excellent job of reviewing Sutent's side effects and you highlighted the potential for yellow skin discoloration. Plus I don't have any signs or symptoms of liver failure; no itching, dark tea- colored urine, acholic stools[10] and my eyes aren't yellow. So kind of 'mellow yellow' I guess." This reference to the song of the same name was probably even more obscure than Mr. Spock's quote. Although I was hoping for a "quite rightly" response, I was almost certain it would not be forthcoming.

"What other side effects have you been experiencing?"

<Bummer. Still, she is an excellent oncology fellow and I'm glad to have her as my doc on this protocol.>

The list of side-effects was long and grew longer[11] as the cycles accrued. Agreeably the yellow skin discoloration and rash did not persist. The side-effects were a significant burden, which temporarily became lighter when the next scan showed significant disease response to the Sutent. That was a good day.

---

[10] Acholic stools are soft, pale, greasy, foul-smelling bowel movements that result from a lack of bile. Bile is a fluid secreted by the liver and discharged into the small intestine where it aids in the digestive process, especially of fats.

[11] The sunitinib side-effects which I experienced included hand-foot syndrome, stomatitis with discrete mouth ulcers, mucositis, epistaxis (nasal bleeding), indigestion, nausea, intestinal cramps and gas, loose stools, rash, yellow skin discoloration, white hair discoloration, decrease in red blood cells, white blood cells and platelets, high blood pressure, headache and dry eyes. Thankfully I did not experience fatigue, one of the more common side- effects of sunitinib.

THIS IS RIDICULOUS – STRIKE ONE
AUTUMN 2005

"What the hell is this?" said the emergency physician, tossing a letter onto my desk in front of me. "We've been fired!"

"What are you talking about?" I replied while picking up the letter.

I began reading and "…Pinnacle Health Hospitals is terminating your current Physician Employment Agreement…" jumped off the page and gave me a "good morning" dope slap. It was early in the morning and although I hadn't yet opened the certified letter at the top of my inbox, I now knew what it said. I opened my letter (Figure 1) and read it to confirm. Yes, I was terminated.

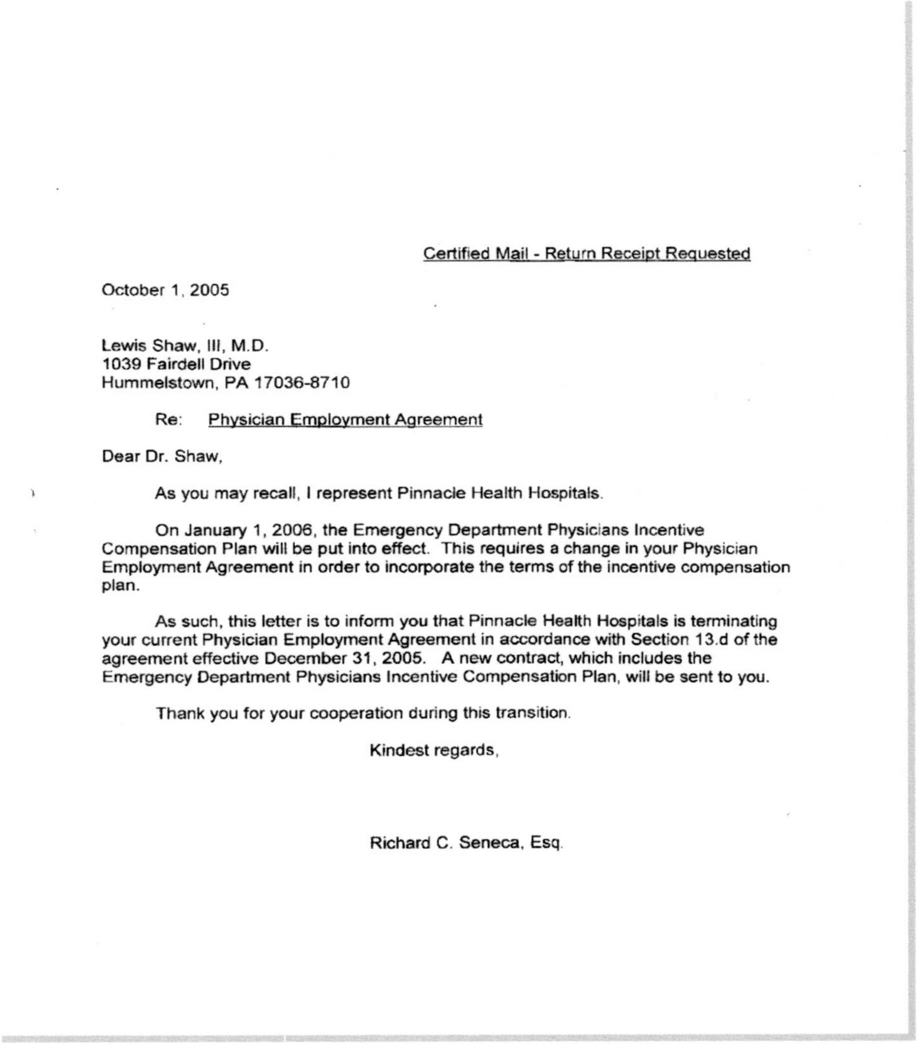

<u>Certified Mail - Return Receipt Requested</u>

October 1, 2005

Lewis Shaw, III, M.D.
1039 Fairdell Drive
Hummelstown, PA 17036-8710

Re: <u>Physician Employment Agreement</u>

Dear Dr. Shaw,

As you may recall, I represent Pinnacle Health Hospitals.

On January 1, 2006, the Emergency Department Physicians Incentive Compensation Plan will be put into effect. This requires a change in your Physician Employment Agreement in order to incorporate the terms of the incentive compensation plan.

As such, this letter is to inform you that Pinnacle Health Hospitals is terminating your current Physician Employment Agreement in accordance with Section 13.d of the agreement effective December 31, 2005. A new contract, which includes the Emergency Department Physicians Incentive Compensation Plan, will be sent to you.

Thank you for your cooperation during this transition.

Kindest regards,

Richard C. Seneca, Esq.

Figure 1

"I don't know what this is about. I'll investigate and let you know."

Before I finished the second sentence he had turned his back and, without another word, was out the door returning to work in the department.

<This is not going to be a good day…Ya think?>

This should be easy to investigate I thought. I'll just phone the appropriate administrator. His administrative assistant answered his line and informed me he wasn't immediately available. I requested he page me at his earliest convenience.

"Can I tell him what this is about?" she asked.

"It's about all the emergency physicians being fired," I replied.

"Oh my," was her startled response.

His page was not long in coming. My call to his direct number was answered promptly.

"Hi, it's Lew," I said.

"Lew, they haven't been fired," he said immediately.

"The letter states 'Pinnacle Health Hospitals is terminating your current Physician Employment Agreement'. There doesn't appear to be another way to interpret that statement."

"But they're going to be getting new contracts."

"Of course, all of our contracts end December 31 and they were expecting the next iteration of their contracts to be revised reflecting the performance incentive plan. However, they weren't expecting to be terminated."

"They weren't," he persisted.

"But, that's what the letter says. Why wasn't I given the opportunity to preview and comment on the letters, or at least a 'heads up' that they were coming?"

Silence.

"Why even send the letters? Just send the new contracts," I concluded.

"The hospital attorney blah, blah, blah…"

I stopped listening.

<This is going to get ugly.>

"... blah, blah."

"Just to be clear, they are going to believe they have been fired because that's what the letter says. You should inform the higher ups."

"Sure."

"Goodbye."

"Goodbye."

As everyone who has or has ever had a job knows, some work days seem longer than others. This one could have been measured in full moons. Quickly I learned my script.

Everyone: "Why were the doctors fired?"

Me: "The administration felt the letters were needed prior to the new physician contracts being sent."

Everyone: "Did you know about the letters?"

Me: "No."

Everyone: "Did you get a letter?"

Me: "Yes."

Everyone who was not an emergency physician: "What's going to happen?"

Me: "The doctors will receive their new contracts to sign."

As that workday crumbled towards its end, my sense that this episode would become ugly was already confirmed. Snippets of conversations and confidential "asides" indicated the majority of the Emergency

Physicians were inclined to retain legal counsel, and since they were all in the same situation, the same legal counsel. At the end of that day three things were true that were not true at its beginning. First, the majority of my staff were angry with me and didn't trust me because I had not informed them they were receiving apparent termination letters. Second, the administration was angry with me and didn't trust me because I hadn't convinced the emergency physicians they weren't being fired and hadn't managed their reaction better. Third, I was seriously considering applying for disability.

The contract issue chafed more and more as autumn progressed. It was a distraction, one which infused the days with more distress than necessary. The emergency physicians had selected an attorney who was uniquely antagonistic toward the hospital and one of the administrators would occasionally state openly that the emergency physicians were threatening to strike. Although it remains unclear to me how someone who has been terminated can threaten to strike, there it is. All of this added to my workload and disease burden.

The side-effects of the sunitinib (Sutent) were increasingly challenging. The protocol specified a cycle as four weeks on drug, taken once daily, then two weeks off drug. The half-life[12] sunitinib is about two days and that of its primary active metabolite is about four days. Consequently the drug was not completely cleared from my body prior to the start of each successive cycle. The side-effects slowly, inexorably worsened as I tallied cycles. Although I experienced a multitude of sunitinib's side effects the hand-foot syndrome, palmar-plantar erythrodysesthesia for fans of formal medical terminology, was the worst. By late autumn 2005 the end of each cycle brought several days of shuffling gait as the push-off for a normal stride was too painful. I wore exam gloves for almost every task. File folder edges felt like a sharp knife edge to my unprotected skin. The list of substances, some obvious in retrospect, which were of no benefit included tea tree oil, PAV ointment, zinc oxide, lanolin oil, ammonium lactate cream, dimethicone, petrolatum and Silvadene. Urea cream was of marginal benefit. Only a cumbersome

[12] Half-life is the time it takes for half of a drug/toxin in one's system to be cleared. Typically after five half-lives an insignificant amount of that substance remains in the body. For example if drug A has a half-life of 24 hours, after five days an insignificant amount of drug A remains in the system. This concept is independent of the amount of a drug/toxin which needs to be present to have an effect. In the case of sunitinib the drug accumulates to a level of 3 to 4 times that of a single dose and the primary active metabolite accumulates to a level of 7 to 10 times that of a single dose.

process enabled me to exercise. Twenty to thirty minutes before exercising I slathered local anesthetic cream (lidocaine/prilocaine) onto the soles of my feet then donned thin cotton socks under athletic socks. The local anesthetic enabled up to 45 minutes of exercise. Immediately upon finishing exercise I doffed my socks and soaked my feet in iced baking soda water; two heaping tablespoons of baking soda dissolved in about a quart of water, add ice, stir, add feet.

It was late in the afternoon of a day during such an interval when the call from our Chief Medical Officer came. Our Chief Medical Officer was a good guy and uncommonly reasonable and thoughtful, two praiseworthy qualities in what, I imagined, was a thankless job.

"Hello, Emergency Department, Lew Shaw. Can I help you?"

"Hi Lew, it's Dana. Can you come over to my office?"

"Sure. Should I bring anything?"

"No."

"Okay, I'll be right over."

"Thanks. Goodbye."

"Bye."

This can only be about the contract issue I thought as I removed my gloves and began the painful ambulation to Dana's office. The accumulating distress from being alone in the middle between the emergency physicians and the administration was becoming exasperating and the situation seemed to be at an impasse.

<This is too problematic. I'll strongly recommend he contract with an Emergency Department physician staffing company to staff the Emergency Departments. I know he's considering it, in fact maybe he's going to tell me he's decided to do just that. It will resolve the issue for me and while the transition is occurring I'll "go out" on disability. Now that's a solid plan! ... What took you so long? … Doesn't really matter, does it? … Not really.>

I felt relieved as I shuffled through an almost empty administrative suite to Dana's office.

"Hi Dana."

"Hi Lew. Come in, have a seat."

"Thanks."

"Can we have our physicians staffing our Emergency Departments come January 1?" he asked, getting immediately to the point.

"Yes," I heard myself say.

<WHAT, you just said what?! That wasn't the plan! Are you nuts?>

"Good," said Dana.

Briefly we discussed the strategy for accomplishing this objective and I was on my way, shuffling painfully back to my office.

<You were done, problem solved! You were out the door without shame! How are you going to pull this off? … Maybe this is that "chemo brain" thing I've heard about… Whatever it is, this is ridiculous!>

"GREEN GRASS AND HIGH TIDES" THE OUTLAWS

If I study for a test the result will be better than if I don't study for that test. Gradually over the years, I had become confident in my test taking ability. Know what material is being surveyed by the test, study the material, prepare for the test, take the test believing that I will pass the test and pass the test. For me the first three steps of the process are essential for having the correct attitude during the test. Consequently, I suspect some of my poor test results (liver biopsy positive for cancer, scans demonstrating tumor progression, blood tests showing liver failure, etc.) could've been prevented were I able to study for those tests.

I needed to pass the American Board of Emergency Medicine (ABEM) recertification exam to maintain ABEM certification and I needed to maintain ABEM certification to retain my job. Almost certainly this would be the last standardized, comprehensive exam I would ever take, the first having been over 40 years prior. However, I would not be able to study or prepare adequately for this exam because of distractions, distractions, distractions. These considerable distractions were related to having a family, being an Emergency Medicine Department Chair and waging war against cancer -- the good, the bad and the ugly. The end result was that I was understudied and felt ill-prepared for the ABEM recertification exam on October 26, 2006. The exam date fell within the active treatment phase of a cycle, at a time I would be experiencing debilitating side-effects of the sunitinib. The conundrum was whether or not to request a drug holiday for the exam. Given my year and a half of experience with sunitinib I knew that a single day off drug would not help. I would need 4 to 5 days off drug prior to the exam in order for the side-effect reduction to be meaningful.

<Not smart to be off drug during an active treatment phase unless medically necessary… It is necessary to pass the test and a drug holiday might be an essential part of your preparation… Don't know that for a fact… No, the future is notoriously difficult to predict… Disease progression… Exam failure… Disease progression… Exam failure…>

My request for a drug holiday was granted.

I had not been truly anxious about a test in a long, long time. I was truly anxious about this test and my anxiety crescendoed during the unfamiliar pre-exam sign in for this computer-based test at a generic testing center. Most of the other examinees were taking other standardized exams. There was a very high level of security with very strict, rigid processes for all aspects of the test, especially for taking a bathroom break. Much to my surprise and relief once I started the test calm washed over me. After all of the fuss this was a test of knowledge and I could take a test. Of course that didn't prevent anxiety from returning after completing the test, immediately after, in the parking lot of the testing center. There were too many questions for which I was not certain of the answer.

The same distractions which prevented proper preparation for the test now attenuated the weighty wait for the test results. Some weeks later I made it home from work early one evening to find the test results had arrived in that day's mail, and to find my wife and son both very anxious for me to open the envelope. They were perplexed not only by my precondition to have "Green Grass and High Tides" playing loudly on the stereo, but especially by my insistence that the opening of the envelope coincide with a particular passage of the song.

I explained that in the spring of 1978 "Green Grass and High Tides" had been playing loudly on the stereo when I opened the envelope containing my Medical College Admission Test (MCAT) results.

They appeared more perplexed. I elaborated; since that episode the results of every standardized test I took were opened to that passage of "Green Grass and High Tides" and that wasn't going to change now, at which point they exchanged a look indicating they had concluded I was nuts. It isn't that I'm superstitious, but in this instance I wanted all the help, real or imagined, that I could get in attaining a passing score of 75 or better. The moment came and I opened the envelope. The distractions had indeed taken their toll. My score was 91, significantly lower than in 1996.

COSMIC BAD LUCK
JANUARY 30, 2007

It was time to go shopping again. It had been more than two years since I had seen an authoritative neuroendocrine cancer specialist. I was approaching two years on the Sutent protocol and although there had been no significant disease progression, side-effects had necessitated a dose reduction. Sutent would not perpetually sustain me. Contingency plans A and B needed to be crystallized. My ongoing review and analysis of the national neuroendocrine cancer landscape led me to seek out Dr. Eugene Woltering, a preeminent neuroendocrine cancer specialist in New Orleans, Louisiana. The "new patient dance" was performed and Stephanie and I were on our way to New Orleans. Although the circumstances were such that the long trip was only overnight, I was delighted to have Steph's company on this segment of my Odyssey. I suspect that having not accompanied me to Houston in 2004, she wanted to hear what the oncologist said directly rather than through my filter. Our six-year-old son, Nate was eager to be in his own house under his grandparents' supervision for two days. Nate was one of the factors in my selection of Dr. Woltering. Having been diagnosed with a rare cancer at the age of 47, I wanted to know if neuroendocrine cancer should be on my list of worries about him. My reading didn't suggest neuroendocrine cancer needed to be added to my list of parental worries, but I was very worried that it might need to be added. It seemed likely Dr. Woltering would provide a definitive, authoritative answer at the current level of understanding.

After an uneventful trip and overnight in New Orleans, we were in Dr. Woltering's office. The office prelude to Dr. Woltering's entrance was mostly routine and familiar except for the map on the wall. In the map had been placed pins corresponding to the locations of his patients' homes; many, many pins. As there was no pin in our hometown's location, we pinned it.

Dr. Woltering did not disappoint.
"Keep doing what you're doing until it stops working. Monitoring needs to include… Next steps to consider include…"

All of the information excellent and important for Stephanie to hear directly from him. However while listening I realized I was in his office for only one reason, to ask 'the question.' Finally an appropriate time came. After taking a breath I began.

"We have a six-year-old son. Given the circumstances and my age do we need to worry about a neuroendocrine tumor developing in him? Are there any genetic implications? How did I get this disease?" I implored.

"Cosmic bad luck," he replied immediately and assertively.

<I'm good with that.>

The cosmos mandates unequal outcomes and there is nothing we can do to change that fundamental aspect of creation. How we respond to that fate is part of our test. Do we do our best to provide equal opportunity, liberty and assistance to one another so each of us can try for her/his best possible outcome, or do we use the inequality of outcome for some nefarious sociopolitical or bureaucratic purpose? But I digress, again. Sorry.

The most important question had been asked and answered, no genetic worries. Time to enjoy that information and push on.

Epilogue

Everyone knows that smoking (marijuana, tobacco, etc.) causes lung cancer. However many people who smoke do not get lung cancer. Everyone gets exposed to the sun, yet not everyone gets skin cancer. We have two lungs, two kidneys, two ovaries or testicles, but cancer develops in only one. These phenomena are explained by the fact that there is an element of randomness involved in the development of cancer. We humans tend to be uncomfortable with randomness playing a role in such an important development in our lives. We would likely be more comfortable if all cancers were caused by a complex interaction between genetics and environment, one factor predetermined and the other potentially controllable. Although disappointing from the perspective of human desire to have control, the cumulative evidence of the last 10 years is conclusive -- many cancers are cosmic bad luck.

THE UNEXPECTED
SUMMER 2007

The formal conclusion of my participation in the Sutent research protocol was being explained. I needed to return 30 days after the last day on drug to be evaluated, have labs and an electrocardiogram (ECG). The conversation was expected, disappointing but expected. I had known for five weeks that my disease had progressed beyond the protocol limit. The conclusive MRI had been performed on day one of my May, 2007 cycle, but I was permitted to complete the cycle in progress. Subsequently May 29, 2007 marked the end of an era, my last day on Sutent, 27 months as a lab rat. The good news was later that summer Fox Chase Cancer Center was opening a phase 3 study of a different drug for neuroendocrine cancer and I would be eligible.

<Another opportunity to be a lab rat.>

Returning to Dr. Alexander's office two weeks later I found him near the ebullient end of his emotional spectrum, at least that portion of his emotional spectrum which I was permitted to see. I suspect his motto was "grab the positive and push on." How else to explain his discussion of disease progression with me?

"You should enjoy feeling good this summer," he began. "After two summers on Sutent you'll be free of side-effects this summer. The preliminary studies of Afinitor have been promising and since Afinitor's mechanism of action is different from Sutent's, it's a very reasonable next move for you. Also the only way you can get the drug is to participate in a trial, as it is not yet approved. Even the timing is excellent. The study won't open at Fox Chase for about two months and that should fit nicely with any washout interval which the protocol will require."

"All true, but it's progressing," I reflexively responded.

"Yes but your total disease burden is less than when you were diagnosed, now what, three years ago? Remember the goal is to keep your ship off the rocks. The disease is not going to get away from us in the next 2 to 3 months."

"Okay, it will feel good to be free of the side- effects," I admitted.

"Enjoy it."

I did, for about three weeks. In addition to the hand-foot syndrome, mucositis, high blood pressure, headaches, whitening of my hair, nausea, indigestion, intestinal cramps and flatus, diarrhea, neutropenia (decreased number of white blood cells), thrombocytopenia (decreased number of platelets), yellow skin, rash and taste disturbance all subsiding; the constant noxious, toxic feeling of the drug's presence in my system was almost completely gone. Consequently it was startling and unnerving to experience an irregular heartbeat. I could feel my heartbeat flip-flopping. My pulse was regularly irregular, every other beat occurring earlier than it should; a 'bigeminal rhythm' for you medical terminology fans. In my 50 years I had never had a heart issue and it was only about two weeks since I had a normal ECG as part of the protocol wrap-up. I was about to step onto the elliptical trainer to exercise when I noticed it.

<M.D. means 'Makes Decisions', so make one! If I call Ron he'll tell me to go to the ER and get an ECG, but that won't really tell why this is happening and what to do. That will mean the inevitable cardiology consult and the rest of the day will be shot. I feel really good, overall better than I've felt since I started the Sutent... Okay, get on the elliptical and start very, very slowly. If you increase your heart rate and the bigeminy resolves, it's probably not serious and you don't need to make a special trip to the hospital. Start extremely slowly. Any lightheadedness or worsening of the pulse you stop and go immediately to the ER. You go directly to the ER, do not pass 'Go', do not collect $200.>

So I got on the elliptical and started slowly, very, very s-l-o-w-l-y. Over the next few minutes I gradually increased my revolutions per minute and my heart rate. I felt fine. A few minutes later and the irregular heartbeat vanished. A perfect, regular pulse returned. I felt even better and I attacked, completing the 30 minute workout with my top end heart rate in the mid-150s.

<YES!>

My heart rate gradually return to normal and the irregular heartbeat did not return.

<YES, YES!>

About two weeks later I was in Dr. Alexander's office to discuss the details of the Afinitor RAD 001 protocol.

"About two weeks ago I had an episode of bigeminy," I said as a prelude to our discussion of the RAD 001 protocol.

"You didn't call," Dr. Alexander replied matter-of-factly.

"It went away with exercise and didn't recur," I said, unsuccessfully attempting to match his 'cool.'

"Okay," he said. "Any questions or concerns about RAD 001?"

"No. I'm convinced that Afinitor is the best next step. Obviously I wish I didn't have to accept a 50% chance of starting on placebo in order to get the drug."

"Not many people have 'participating in a placebo-controlled phase 3 study of a drug for metastatic cancer' on their bucket list," he deadpanned.

"I am amazed that a drug company is able to get insurance companies to subsidize its research (Appendix A, excerpt from the RAD 001 protocol consent). According to the protocol my insurance carrier will be billed for labs, imaging studies, office visits and even medications to manage side-effects of the Afinitor! I presume I'll need to pay deductibles and co-pays, so in effect I'm paying to be a lab rat! How does that happen?"

"For phase 3 studies the drug companies have successfully argued that the care which you just mentioned would be routine care for you if you weren't participating in the study and consequently should be paid for by insurance and/or the patient. Anything else?"

"I'm having some logistical difficulties scheduling my screening colonoscopy so I haven't had it yet."

"Okay, let me know when you've had it. I'm glad you're doing so well."

"Thanks. See you soon."

I returned to enjoying the summer. It was the best I had felt during a summer since the summer of 2003. I had adapted to two situations which would have been inconceivable had I considered them in my younger years, being on call 24 hours a day, seven days a week and having incurable metastatic cancer.

My workload as Chair stabilized that summer at 40 to 45 hours every week and there were no overwhelming weeks. I was able to play in the one golf tournament which I had entered annually since 1996, the Hershey Country Club Member-Guest Tournament. The tournament was becoming more precious with each passing year. I played with the same partner, a life-long friend, and we thoroughly enjoyed the two and a half days of friendly competition. Just us in a golf cart.

For two and a half days each year adult responsibilities did not exist and we were young again. The semblance of a routine was developing during the treatment hiatus, when one day my dear, sweet wife said,

"You're not dead yet."

<Huh?>

"What I mean is it seems you're doing well and there is no reason to believe you won't continue to do well," she explained.

"That is the situation as I understand it," I responded still not sure where this unexpected conversation was going.

"You're in this drug-free period and we don't know if that will ever happen again. So, I think we should take this opportunity to have some sperm frozen," she said starting to get to the point.

<?!>

"Then if you're stable on this new drug and you continue to do well, we can use the frozen sperm for in vitro fertilization[13] and have another child," she concluded.

"Sure," I said, naïvely relieved the conversation had such a simple destination.

[13] In Vitro Fertilization is a process in which ova (eggs) harvested from the woman's ovaries are placed in a medium to which sperm are added. The resulting fertilized eggs (zygotes) are placed in the uterus and allowed to develop to term.

"KEEP PUSHIN"
REO SPEEDWAGON

Although, in the moment, days can seem slow, when seen retreating in the rearview mirror years seem fast, even years on chemo.

<How does the brain do that?... Don't know, but there must be a neurophilosophical[14] explanation… Okay, but how did I get from counting cycles to counting years?... Come on, you know that.>

Being able to count years is part luck. Metastatic cancer is an incredibly complex disease with scores of intertwined and interconnected biochemical pathways. Each one of us has incredibly complex genetics and is unique. Consequently one's response, or lack thereof to a treatment and the side-effects experienced are unique to that individual, and that is before considering the performance of any proceduralists (surgeon, interventional radiologist) involved! Equality of outcome is not possible and each patient's outcome is partially determined by luck.

Being able to count years is part good decision-making. Good decision-making requires the absence of bad information; which sounds simple, but isn't always so (consider laboratory error, incorrect interpretation of CT/MRI scans, false claims by purveyors of alternative therapies). Good decision-making requires excellent input from your medical team. Good decision-making isn't about one's intelligence, education or professional success. Even an incredibly successful creative genius can make bad treatment decisions[15]. Consideration of your specific constitution and situation are of paramount importance in your decision-making. It is

---

[14] Neurophilosophy is the study of how the brain makes the conscious mind; the central concept being that the mind and the brain are one, not functionally separate yet structurally coexistent. While certainly an implicit part of the neurosciences for hundreds of years, correct use of the term by medical students in a U.S. medical college neuroscience lecture hall is documented in April, 1980 (Appendix B, author's lecture notes). We concluded that if we were clever enough connect the dots and coin the term, then so were many other medical students in many other medical college lecture halls.

[15] Steve Jobs by Walter Isaacson, Simon & Schuster, 2011.

scary, but the decisions are ultimately yours.

Being able to count years is part good medical care and taking care of one's self. Good medical care is self-explanatory. The design of the human organism is incomprehensibly elegant. Every organ system is fully, completely integrated with all of the other organ systems. Nothing exists in isolation. The significance of this integration is that the cancer patient should attend to and maintain other organ systems while focusing on the cancer; exercise, preventative dental care and hygiene, blood pressure monitoring and control as needed, exercise, proper diet and nutrition, blood sugar control, smoking cessation, routine eye exams, exercise, screening mammograms and colonoscopies, and so on.

Being able to count years is part not thinking about years, but about choosing your attitude toward each day. Each and every day all effort should be directed toward making that day the best day possible, repeat that six times and you will have had the best week possible, repeat that 51 times and you will have had the best year possible; and… you… keep… pushing… on.

I pushed on. Two weeks into the RAD 001 protocol (October, 2007) I knew I was on placebo, no side- effects. Although I knew there was a 50-50 chance that placebo would be my initial treatment, here I was with disease progression and no active treatment while waiting for the next scan. Occasionally I tried to convince myself I might be on the active drug, going so far as to embellish lingering side-effects of the Sutent which I had discontinued five months prior, but I knew I was taking placebo. The circumstances were unsettling and encumbered the days during the two and a half months until my next scan.

At my January 9, 2008 clinic appointment the Fox Chase treatment team entered and left one by one. After the nurse exited Dr. E. entered, smiling. Providing the usual disclaimer that the radiologist's official measurements and interpretation were pending, he said the MRI appeared to show mild improvement. Next was the protocol nurse Brenda, also smiling. After confirming that Dr. E. had already seen me, she reiterated their overall impression of mild improvement. Brenda said she would forward the official measurements the next day.

<How did that happen on placebo?... Maybe you're not on placebo… However it happened, stable is good, improvement is better!>

January 10th came and went with no follow-up.

My pager vibrated at about 4 PM on Friday, January 11. Recognizing the area code, I had that sudden sinking feeling and felt hot all over. I called the number and the phone was answered, "Hello, Dr. E.'s office." I was certain that the news was bad. The oncology fellow and/or protocol nurse typically conveyed good news, but he alone would deliver bad news, which he did. The measured disease progression required the study code be broken to determine whether I was in the placebo arm or the active drug arm. He said he would contact me Monday with the information.

<Shit, shit, shit! What if I'm on the active drug?... Focus, you know you're not... But what if I am? I'll be dropped from the study and contingency plan A hasn't been defined… FOCUS!>

About a half hour later I was again paged to Dr. E.'s office. I was given the expected news, I had been on placebo. I was to begin the active drug, Afinitor (everolimus) immediately. It was being overnight shipped to my house and I should begin taking it tomorrow. The next day the Afinitor arrived and shortly thereafter so did the side-effects. While the side-effects I experienced from Afinitor were not as plentiful nor as severe as those associated with Sutent, there were no "off drug" days in the RAD 001 protocol. Afinitor stabilized my disease and by early 2009 I counted five years from diagnosis and one year on Afinitor.

Stephanie also had counted one year on Afinitor.

"You've been stable for a year on this drug," she commented one day. "I think it's time to use the frozen sperm for IVF[16] and try to have another child."

<If she is brave enough to have a child with a husband in my condition, I can't be the weak link in this partnership.>

"Sure," I replied, instantly having a dramatically new perspective on the simple decision to have sperm frozen.

[16] IVF – In Vitro Fertilization is a process in which ova (eggs) harvested from the woman's ovaries are placed in a medium to which sperm are added. The resulting fertilized eggs (zygotes) are placed in the uterus and allowed to develop to term.

AN UNEXPECTED QUESTION
MARCH, 2009

Emergency Departments (EDs) are an easy target for criticism. Everyone either perceives they have had, or knows someone who reports having had a negative ED patient experience. Everyone in every Hospital and Medical Staff Department has had, or knows someone who reports having had a negative interaction at its ED interface. Every experienced Emergency Department chair understands the following metaphor describes the framework within which the job must be performed: You work in the ultimate societal fishbowl. Everyone can urinate in your water and everyone can criticize you for having yellow water. Keeping the water as clean as possible was a big part of my job. Every day there were multiple ongoing interdepartmental issues to address. In addition to ongoing issues, new issues added to each day's challenge. Consequently when approached by a hospital or medical staff colleague my mind typically flicked to any ongoing issue with that person or their department. So it was one day when I was approached by the chair of Orthopedic Surgery while in passing. I had known the chair for about 25 years. We became acquainted because our residency training coincided and we had played together on a competitive softball team for several years.

He responded to my greeting with, "Can I ask you a question?"

"Sure Ron," I replied, thinking he was going to ask about an Orthopedics billing issue of significant concern, which I was investigating.

"Aren't you supposed to be dead?"

"I guess it depends on who you ask."

Thereafter "Aren't you supposed to be dead?" has been an occasional greeting from Ron. Confidentially I enjoy trying to conjure a new, pithy response each time he poses the question.

NOT THAT BRAVE AND NOT VERY SMART

During the Second World War my father was a tail gunner in a U.S. Army Air Corps B-17 bomber. Once, many years ago I asked dad how he came to be in the Army Air Corps. He told me that all of the healthy males knew they would be drafted upon graduation from high school and probably were destined for combat, so he enlisted in the Air Corps rather than risk being drafted into another branch of the military.

When I asked, 'Why the Air Corps?' he replied that they ate better and if he was going to die, it would only hurt for a short while. When I was little I wore his leather flight helmet a lot and still remember the peculiar smell of the rubber oxygen mask. I was curious about the whole undertaking and asked about his personal experience a few times during my childhood years.

He would not discuss the particulars of his service with me and I came to respect his silence on the topic. I sensed his reluctance was based on a significant event, not something heroic or profound such as surviving a German prisoner of war camp as did one of my uncles, but something significant to him nonetheless.

On a few occasions over the years I asked older relatives about Dad's Army Air Corps service. The little information I accrued indicated Dad's crew flew Air-Sea rescue in the southeastern U.S. region. He was transferred to a B-29 bomber crew in the Pacific Theater of operations and was in transit to join that crew when the war ended. Eventually I let go my curiosity.

One day I saw a newspaper announcement that a restored B-17 bomber was to be on display at a nearby airport. It wasn't the first time a restored aircraft was on display at that airport, but this was a B-17 and I had the day off work. My plan was to ask Dad to go for a ride without supplying details and surprise him with the exhibit. (If the reader senses this episode is not going to end well for me, you are correct.) As we entered the airport and drove to the parking area a hanger blocked the aircraft from view so the element of surprise was maintained. My curiosity had returned and I was excited. Surely after the passing of so many years he would tell me about his service. As we walked around the hanger and the plane came into view my gaze locked on Dad's face so I would remember his expression. When Dad saw the B-17 his face froze in a peculiar expression which seemed to be a combination of dread and anger. He remained silent as we approached the plane. In the few minutes before the docent began his presentation Dad's expression did not change and he did not say a word. The guide was less than five minutes into his narrative when dad said grimly and quietly, "That's not how we did it. I'm going back to the car." Despite his departure I was going to listen to the presentation and wait my turn to go inside the B-17. My stubbornness comes in equal portions from my parents. After a seemingly interminable wait I climbed into the B-17.

<Front-yes, middle-yes, time to get to the tail.>

I began to crawl along the narrow conduit toward the tail.

<Wow this is a very tight fit, no space to maneuver… Remind you of anything dumb ass, like maybe a MRI gantry?>

The epiphany was profound. I squeezed into the tail gunner's position and tried to imagine it in a different place and time.

After a silent and very uncomfortable ride home my curiosity remained unsatisfied, but I knew I would never again approach the topic with Dad.

COSMIC GOOD LUCK

Long before scrapbooking evolved from a hobby into an art form Dad scrapbooked one event, our 1971 trip to and trek through the Philmont Scout Ranch in Cimarron, New Mexico. At fourteen I was the youngest member of the crew and probably no better than an "even money" bet to finish the trek.

I was a skinny 100 pounder and when we left base camp my backpack weighed 42 pounds. I was not very tough physically or mentally. The trip was of great importance to Dad, an Assistant Scoutmaster and he has talked about it many times in the 45 years since the trip.

The scrapbook is meticulous, a zippered leather binder which I have perused many times over the decades. One day I borrowed the scrapbook to show to a crewmate. Prior to meeting with my former crewmate I opened the scrapbook to enjoy the memory of a successfully completed trek.

The binder's contents were astonishing. While the binder was identical in appearance to the Philmont scrapbook, this was a scrapbook of Dad's life. Although I knew I was invading Dad's privacy I could not stop examining its contents. Certainly I was not meant to see this while he was alive. One item in particular was overwhelming (Figure 1.). After copying that one item I closed and sealed the scrapbook. The next day I returned it to Dad with a sincere apology.

"Dad, I don't think you intended for me to see this. Sorry."

The path to earthly existence is extremely narrow and surrounded by chance.

2

THE PANTHER CUB

Official newspaper of the Johnstown Center of the University of Pittsburgh. Cypress Avenue School, Johnstown, Pa. Entered as third class matter at Johnstown Postoffice, March 7, 1936, under Section 453½, P. L. & R.

Editorial Staff: Jack Bernet and Ben Morrow, co-editors; Kay Faulkner, feature editor; Robert Worley, photographer; Dan Bowers, Charles R. Colbert, Jr., R. G. Gordon, Stella-Marie Gorgon, Dean Jobe, Paul Jones, Edward A. Mish, Regina Patterson, Jacob Schnegg, Gerald L. Sharpe, Mary Lois Sheridan, Don Thompson, Ed Turek, J. M. Wheeler. Room Mate

Sports Staff: Ben Morrow, Howard Cummings, Jacob Schnegg, Ed Turek.

Business Staff: John Lewis, Harry Morrow and Tom Berriman.

Circulation: Irene Nagg.

PRINTED BY SCHUBERT PRESS, INC.— 4—JOHNSTOWN, PENNA.

B. M.

Center Student Cheats Death

There was more than an eighty-cent meal awaiting Lewis Shaw as he walked into the Ohio Street restaurant the other night.

There was a story of death—death in which Lew might have been an unwilling victim.

Lew, a Pre-dent sophomore, dropped into the resaurant as usual for his evening meal. Suddenly someone shouted his name.

"Shaw!"

"Clark! Clark Hauer! What are you doing here?"

And so two former GI buddies met.

It was during the eager conversation that followed that Shaw discovered how he had unknowingly cheated death four years ago.

The story began at Drew Field, Florida, where an anxious group of young airforce men in a B-17 squadron were learning the tactics of aerial warfare.

Shaw was tail gunner on one of the B-17's. He, along with members of the crew, had spent countless hours making assimilated attacks, firing at tow targets, practicing air to sea rescue work, and flying at high altitudes in order to get accusotmed to wearing oxygen masks.

Before many weeks had passed, the young fliers had learned their job well; however, one thing was wrong. All during the training period Shaw and the pilot had not been able to get along very well with one another. The result was that Shaw said was, "What ever ferred to a B-29 squadron.

From Drew Field, Shaw's former outfit shipped out to the Pacific theater, where they were to be assigned from air to sea duty.

That was the last Shaw heard of his old outfit until the other night. Hauer had shipped out on one of the B-17's, and of course, after greeting his buddy the first thing that Shaw s aid was, What ever happened to my old crew?"

"Didn't you hear about it?" asked Hauer. "They were lost somewhere in the Pacific. No one ever knew exactly what happened to them. They just disappeared while on a routine mission."

"Wow!" said Shaw, putting his hand to his forehead, "I'm glad now I got kicked off that crew."

Just because of a clash of personalities, Shaw had escaped death in the Pacific Ocean, and it took him four years to discover the fact.

Figure 1
Cosmic Good Luck

THIS IS RIDICULOUS – STRIKE TWO
OCTOBER, 2009

I was getting a few looks from the other passengers, but not many. Given the circumstances I was bewildered that no one else was wearing a face mask. The influenza epidemic was creating havoc for the medical community. This epidemic was occurring much earlier than the typical flu season having first appeared in the U.S. in April, 2009. The virus spread rapidly throughout the world and in June, 2009 the World Health Organization raised the global pandemic alert to 6, its highest level. Our preparations for the influx of patients related to this flu epidemic were extensive and included a patient care trailer outside each of our Emergency Departments, in order to keep as many flu patients as possible from entering the hospitals.

There was no vaccine to protect against the circulating strain of the virus. The virus was highly contagious and there was no significant pre-existing immunity in the population. It was particularly dangerous to infants, individuals with pre-existing lung or heart diseases, pregnant patients and those who were immunocompromised. Stephanie was in the eighth month of pregnancy and, in an effort to recruit Emergency Physicians, my immunocompromised body was on an airplane traveling to Boston for the American College of Emergency Physicians annual Scientific Assembly.

Yes, you read correctly, Stephanie was pregnant. By way of in vitro fertilization her pregnancy was a triumph of technology. It was also a triumph of faith, courage and determination over fear and doubt. While we both knew the potential for a widow-with-two-small-children scenario, we chose not to discuss it; not because of denial, but because of faith we had chosen the correct path. Significant nausea and vomiting complicated the early portion of the pregnancy for Stephanie. Growing trepidation complicated the entire pregnancy for me. Concern for her health increased as it became clear this strain of influenza was decidedly more deadly for pregnant women. Additionally, the realization that I had chosen the responsibility of another child with a very difficult implicit goal became starker as the pregnancy progressed.

<This is ridiculous! I'm flying into a large population center where thousands of travelers are congregating in a convention center. No chance for exposure to the flu there... You dumb ass, it's very unlikely you're going to recruit even one doc at this event.>

The effort was expected. Recruiting was one of the Chair's essential duties and resolving our Emergency Physician shortage was required. We had been short-staffed Emergency Physicians for five months despite an intense recruiting effort and, with no candidates in sight, there seemed no alternative to personally attending the annual Emergency Medicine Residents Association (EMRA) Job Fair associated with the Scientific Assembly. I had thoroughly enjoyed every one of the many previous Scientific Assemblies which I attended, but not this one as I endured constant concern about the flu. No one was wearing a face mask in the convention center and remaining several feet away from all people at all times was not possible. 'Keep your eye glasses on, hands clean and don't touch your face' was my mantra. It's unknowable if any of the precautions helped, but I felt better going through the motions. I sat or stood so that no one was behind me in the lecture halls, I did not shake hands except as required at the job fair and if someone coughed I found another bathroom.

The evening of the job fair arrived. As this was the first time I attended the EMRA Job Fair in any capacity I didn't know what to expect as an exhibitor. I completed set up of the display table and stood waiting for a prospective colleague.

<This is a really nice event. Well thought out. It's cool that small hospitals have the same size display table as large contract groups and it's divided into geographic regions for efficiency. Interesting that the Northeast region has the sparsest crowd given that we are in Boston.>

I continued to stand waiting for a prospective colleague. A senior resident stopped by the table to say, "I'm from Pennsylvania but I'm going to be working in Boston. The professional environment in Pennsylvania is awful." Shortly after she departed another senior resident stopped at the table.
"Pennsylvania?" he started. "Does your organization have any facilities in Maryland or Virginia? The practice environment in Pennsylvania is terrible."

<UGH! Our governor is a horse's ass.>

A grand total of six individuals stopped at my exhibit that evening. Two would come to Harrisburg for an interview. As I began to pack up the display materials, I started thinking about getting home where I perceived my flu risk would be less. After arriving home I would need to avoid contact with Stephanie and Nate for a few days in case I was incubating/carrying the flu. I then discouragingly thought it might be best to avoid contact with them for the duration of the epidemic, as I would be at the hospital daily.

The morning after arriving home I returned to work.

"Did you have any success?" queried Carla, our Emergency Department's (ED) Administrative Assistant, who was as eager as I to resolve our Emergency Physician shortage.

"I think we have a chance of getting one," I responded. "Her fiancé will be doing an ophthalmology residency at the Hershey Medical Center, so she's definitely coming to the area and I think there's a chance she will want to work here. Whoever gets her will be very fortunate because she is going to be an All-Star."

"You know that, how?" Carla gently challenged.

"Sometimes I just know. There were 28 candidates for the ED Administrative Assistant position, but when I met you I simply knew you were the right person to manage the department's logistics. Somehow I know she is going to be a wonderful Emergency Physician. If she does come here to work and I don't come down with the flu and die, the entire disagreeable trip will have been worthwhile."

[Thank you Lindsay.]

"MY SILVER LINING"
FIRST AID KIT

"How was your appointment?" I was asking Stephanie about her final prenatal visit before the scheduled Cesarean section (C-section) delivery.

"Fine. No problems, but one odd thing happened," she replied.

"What was that?"

"The nurse was getting me ready for the doctor's exam and she said 'So, you're having a boy.' "

"What did you say?"

"Not as far as I know."

Very early in the pregnancy we decided not to learn the gender of the baby. We had known our son's gender many weeks before his birth and decided this time to let the gender be a surprise at birth. The suspense had been fun and we enjoyed speculating about the baby's gender.

"Sounds like she let it slip. I don't know how they designate the charts or patients who don't want to know the gender, but I suspect on rare occasions the information slips because in the office the gender of the baby is known and many patients want to know the gender. Unless she's deliberately trying to mislead us."

Two or three mornings later, shortly after waking up, Stephanie said, "I had a vivid dream last night, that it's a boy."

"I guess we better decide on a boy's name," I reflexively responded.

We focused on selecting a name from our short list of potential boy names and by the time for the early-morning drive to the hospital for the C-section delivery we had decided on a name for our son.

The day my son Nate was born in January, 2001 remains one of the five worst days of my life, number four to be exact, but that's another story.

This delivery day was immeasurably better. All was going according to schedule. Stephanie was comfortable and sedated. There were no complications, unexpected events or tense moments. I was about to become an elated, joyful dad! The incisions were made and in short order the head was delivered. After a brief delay to manage the umbilical cord wrapped around the baby's neck, the shoulders were delivered. Then the bottom popped out.

"It's a girl!" I exclaimed, certainly sounding dumbfounded.

"What?" Stephanie said through her drug-induced delirium. She was not able to see our daughter because of the surgical drapes.

"It's a girl!" I repeated.

"You're kidding."

"No, I'm pretty sure."

About that time the neonatologist started narrating her examination of our daughter, convincing us that we were indeed the parents of a healthy girl, not a boy as expected. A healthy girl, but without a name since "Logan" had not been on our short list of girl names.

A day and a half later the short list of girl names was whittled down to "Maggie", a blessing beyond words and my silver lining (Figure 1).

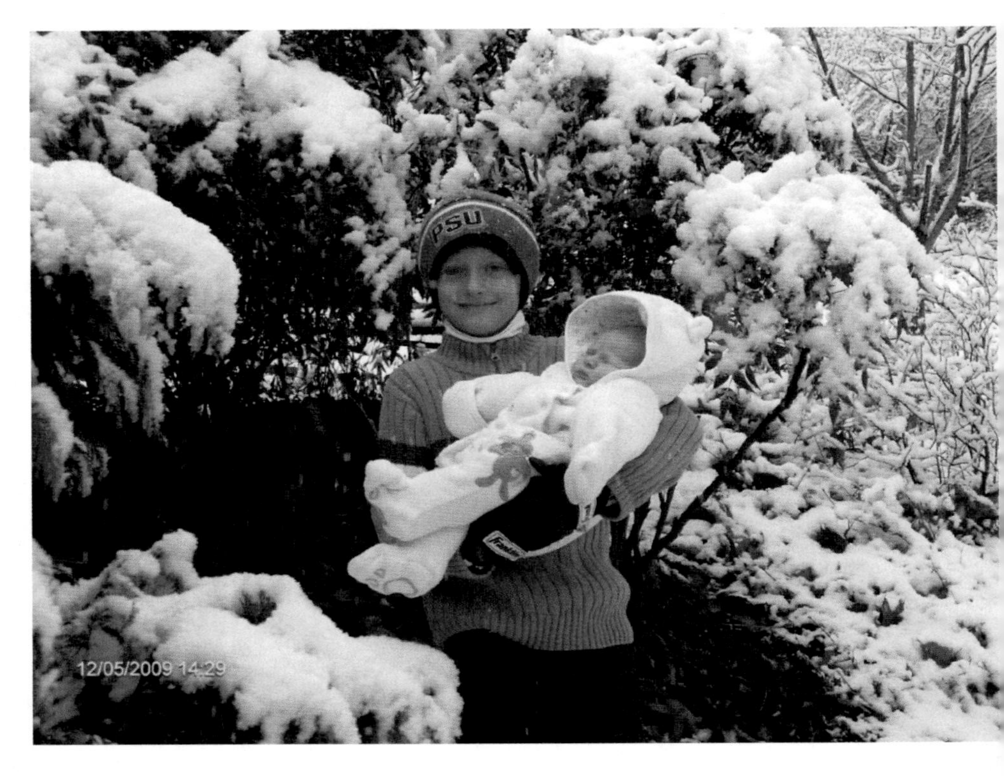

Figure 1
"My Silver Lining"

I WON'T DO THAT AGAIN

MARCH, 2010

"What happened to you?" asked Ron noticing the tightly cinched golf glove on my right hand, the fourth and fifth fingers of which were taped together. Ron, our Chair of Orthopedic Surgery at PinnacleHealth had been a trusted colleague for a quarter of a century. The question was begged as I was walking toward the Medical Staff dining room for lunch and not toward the first tee.

"I broke my fifth metacarpal[17] skiing," I replied not providing details.

"Let me see," he said instantly.

"Ron, while I appreciate your concern I know you're very busy and this is just a fifth metacarpal fracture. It will be okay."

"Let me see it," he repeated.

Thinking the quickest way to be about my business would be to let him examine my hand, I removed the glove.

"When did you do this?" Ron asked as he began to examine my hand.

"Last weekend," I replied.

"How did you do it?"

"Skiing."

"How skiing?"

"I fell off a rail and my hand was still clenched around the pole when I landed on it."

<Fool, trying to ski a rail for the first time at the age of 53… Just trying

[17] The fifth metacarpal is the bone in the hand at the base of the little finger.

to keep up with Nate for a little while longer… You should have known it would end badly!… I did ski the rail twice successfully before crashing… Dumb Ass, you're lucky you weren't hurt worse… Ok, ok I won't do that again.>

"Make a fist," Ron instructed continuing his evaluation. "You jackass it's shortened," he said referring to the knuckle at the base of my little finger, "You've lost length. This needs to be fixed."

"It's only about 1/4 inch shorter and I'm not a surgeon, so my hand doesn't need to be perfect," I said already trying to avoid a trip to the operating room.

"It's your right hand. Are your x-rays in the system?" asked Ron gaining momentum.

"It hasn't been x-rayed. I don't want to take the time."

"Come upstairs. We'll look at it under fluoro[18]. It will only take a minute."

Up to the second floor we went, into the operating suite's (OR) hallways.

"Wait here," Ron instructed, "I'll get the fluoro unit."

Two minutes later we were looking at my right hand under fluoroscopy (Figure 1).

[18] Fluoroscopy is the use of a fluoroscope unit to view x-ray images in real time.

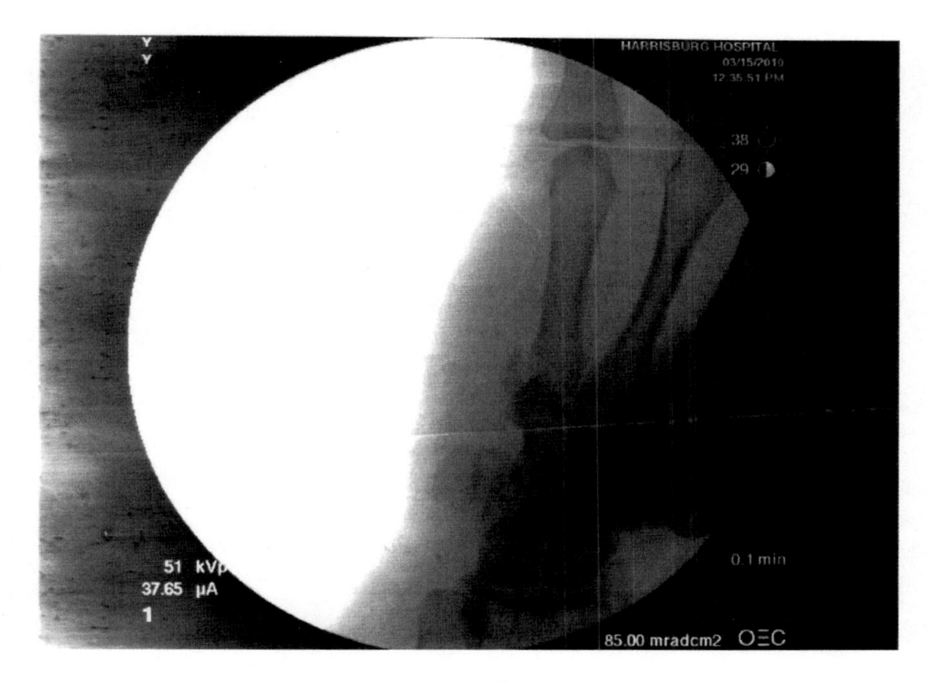

Figure 1
Fractured Fifth Metacarpal

"How cool is this, two Chairs in the OR hallway using the fluoro unit?"

"Pretty cool Ron, pretty cool."

"Okay call my secretary and get yourself scheduled," he said while shutting down the fluoroscope.

It having been impressed upon me that my fracture needed to be fixed in the operating room and that the surgery needed to be done soon, as a few days had already passed since the injury, I was finally able to get back to work.

I hadn't intended to have anyone evaluate my hand, yet now I had a firm recommendation from our Chair of Orthopedics to have surgery. What if I did need surgery to have a stable hand? I called longtime friend and orthopedic surgeon, Bob, and explained the situation. He suggested I get a full set of x-rays, which he could review and then recommend treatment. I also contacted my protocol nurse at Fox Chase Cancer

Center (FCCC) to determine how the proposed surgery would be affected by the RAD-001 protocol and to learn about any prior patient experience with placement of orthopedic hardware while on the protocol.

According to the FCCC investigators zero patients at any study location had undergone surgical treatment of a fracture with placement of orthopedic hardware while on the study drug. As I could not afford losing two, half days of work to have surgery and I didn't want to be the first patient to have orthopedic hardware placed while taking Afinitor, I was seeking support from Bob for a decision not to have surgery.

Fortunately Bob thought I would have a stable hand without surgery. Consequently I did not have surgery to repair the fracture and my hand is fine.

[Thanks Bob!]

"SIMPLE MAN"
LYNRYD SKYNRYD
JUNE 17, 2011

"Mom's dead," I said.

"I'll be right there," my sister Beth instantly replied.

"No, don't," I responded, hoping it was firmly enough to dissuade her.

"Are you sure?"

"Yes, don't come here."

<No reason for you to see her like this.>

"Okay, I'll call Dad."

"Thanks."

"Love you."

"Love you, too."

My sister and I had alternated the vigil at Mom's deathbed for the preceding couple of days when it became obvious she was terminal and very near death. We discussed how Mom expressed guilt about her father dying alone, none of his five daughters in attendance. We were determined not to let that happen to Mom. Dad couldn't participate. After 60 years together, he simply could not endure her earthly end.

Because of logistics our vigil wasn't absolutely continuous. There had been rare, brief gaps in our coverage. Mom died during a 15 minute gap. Maybe it was to assuage the presumed guilt, but as I started to walk from the nurses' station to my mom's room one of the staff commented it seemed like she had been waiting to be alone to "let go." The nurse assured me she had seen it before.

Mom died of idiopathic pulmonary fibrosis, not "Failure to Thrive" which was written on the death certificate[19]. Not to diminish in any way the suffering associated with any other disease, but idiopathic pulmonary fibrosis (IPF) is a cruel, horrible disease. IPF is about being unable to breathe and when you can't breathe NOTHING else matters. It is an inexorably progressive, wasting disease, which kills slowly. The only treatment in 2011 was a lung transplant and at her age Mom wasn't going to consider that therapy. Even if eligible she would not deprive a younger person in need of the scarce resource.

How many times had the nurses and I left family members alone with the body of their loved one? Now I was alone with the body of my mom. Items bobbed to the surface of the torrent in my mind.

<Sorry I wasn't here Mom, but I know you probably did want it that way… You didn't get to die at home though, Dad wasn't going to permit that. Probably the only time in 60 years with Dad when you didn't get your way… It was simple for you and you determined it should be simple for me. "You should help people directly, like a minister or a doctor," you told me near the end of my sophomore year of college. Like I was going to become a research chemist after that… I still chuckle about the invitation for immediate family members to tour the cadaver lab during my first year of medical school. The same wild horses that could not have dragged Dad into the lab could not have kept you out… You made sure I didn't confuse "simple" with "easy"… You taught me that sometimes the silver lining is very small and hard to find, but here and now it's massive; you won't have to bury me… You had a good sense of humor. Too bad you were often ashamed of it… I'll always miss you. Love you. Thanks, Mom.>

Time to go and be with Dad. Worst day ever.

---

[19] The cause of death is the process that is primarily responsible for that individual's demise (heart attack, multiple traumatic injuries, etc.), as differentiated from the manner of death which is the way that death occurs (natural, accidental, homicide, suicide, undetermined). The vast majority of deaths are natural, in which case the treating physician may determine the cause of death and complete the death certificate, at least in Pennsylvania. Thus in the majority of natural deaths there is not a thorough coroner's investigation or autopsy. Understanding the process and having completed hundreds of death certificates in my career, it is important to realize that any study, analysis, abstraction or exercise which makes any conclusion about actual causes of death based on death certificates as completed by the treating physician is almost certainly bogus.

A MOMENT IN TIME

FRIDAY, AUGUST 26, 2011
5:20 – 5:30 PM

It gets real quiet back here after everyone leaves, I mused. "Back here" was the small Department of Emergency Medicine office suite. In a cul-de-sac behind two sets of card access doors no one could know if I was there, and anyone looking from the outside colonnade in through the reception area window would notice only the baseline safety lighting of our tiny reception area.

<NOW, round through the department one final time before closing up for the day. Should I turn right out of the office suite and start my rounds via the waiting room, finishing in the back of the department and returning to the office via the main hospital lobby; or the reverse? No, go through the main lobby and start in the back of the department.>

As I walked in to the lobby I saw Dr. Ron Alexander entering the hospital through the main doors. After greeting me, he asked with a trace of sarcasm if the much-delayed ED construction project was complete. I was pleased to inform him that construction was complete and offered him a tour. He hesitated for a second and I knew that he really didn't have time for tour. Nonetheless he said, "Show me" and we started. We finished our brisk tour and he said before heading home he needed to go upstairs to arrange for an uninsured patient's post-discharge chemo from a pharmaceutical company.

The next morning while rowing, Ron suffered a cardiac arrest and subsequently died.

Creation occasionally speaks to the individual. Being centered and receptive increases the chance of hearing and thus receiving the blessing offered when creation speaks. Not hearing or choosing to ignore creation's message results in lost opportunity. If I had not listened and not exited the office at that moment, by that route I would have missed Ron and my last memory of Ron would not be that of a cherished colleague extending himself for the benefit of his patient.

[Kim, I'm very sorry for taking those five minutes from you.]

THIS IS RIDICULOUS – STRIKE THREE

FEBRUARY 27–MARCH 4, 2012

<This is delightful. No pager, no worries.>

We had arrived in Key West, Florida earlier that day, our first family vacation in two and a half years. Although I wanted to assign my job the entire blame for the long interval between vacations, it would not have been accurate. Our daughter, Maggie was high energy and high maintenance, so why let that challenge blemish a family vacation. Better to wait until she matured into a better traveling companion. Accurately it was a family vacation. Travelling with the four of us was my dad and we were meeting cousins in Key West. We were getting ready for an early dinner when my phone rang.

<Why didn't I turn that off?!>

"Hi, Lew Shaw."

"Hi Lew, it's Christian." Christian was one of my colleagues in the Emergency Department.

"What's up?"

"You need to call Edie. She thinks you've been exposed to H. Flu[20]."

Edie was the department's Special Projects Manager. Among her many duties and responsibilities was the follow-up of body fluid cultures which the lab reported to contain bad germs.

"But I haven't seen a patient since Friday. It's Monday!"

"Sorry. Still, you should call her," he concluded.

"Thanks, goodbye."

---

[20] H. Flu. – Haemophilus Influenza is a species of bacteria which causes serious infections including pneumonia, bacteremia and meningitis. Not to be confused with the Influenza virus which causes the flu.

“Goodbye.”

I hung up and dialed Edie’s number.

“Hello, Edie B., Emergency Department can I help you?”

“Hi Edie, it’s Lew. I understand you’re looking for me.”

“Lew, sorry to bother you. I know you’re on vacation, but according to the chart you saw a patient and her culture is growing H. Flu. Her name is ____”

“That was three days ago!” I said starting to recall the details of the patient encounter. The patient was an elderly, chronically ill, nonverbal female who resided in an extended care facility. The patient was initially evaluated by a mid-level practitioner who requested I evaluate the patient because the patient’s medical situation was complex and the patient was sick.

“I know,” Edie replied apologetically, “but the lab just called.”

<Immunocompromised and exposed to H. Flu. Three days ago, three days ago! Three days in the wind, this is ridiculous!>

“Presuming you were using standard precautions, you need to have been within three feet of the patient for ten or more minutes to be considered ‘exposed.’ Do you think you were?” Edie asked.

I wore a mask. Yes, definitely I had a mask on the entire time I was in her room I thought as my mental replay of the patient encounter came into focus.

“Edie, I wasn’t that close for that long. She was sick and it was obvious she needed admitted. Also, I wore a mask.”

“You’re sure?”

“Yes.”

“Then you don’t fulfill the criteria for being ‘exposed.’ That’s good.”

"Are the rest of the staff who took care of her okay?"

"Yes, they've all been contacted."

"Good. How is she doing?"

"She was in the ICU."

"Wow, sounds like she got sicker. Thanks for tracking me down."

"Just doing my job. Enjoy your vacation. Tell Steph I said 'Hi'."

"Will do. Bye."

"Goodbye."

I turned off my phone.

<You got a little frantic there… Obviously this vacation is needed… Obviously>

The next three days, Tuesday, Wednesday and Thursday were a totally joyful family interlude. Friday was spent riding jet skis around Key West (Figure 1). After returning from our jet ski jaunt, I felt very itchy all over, which I attributed to a never-before-used brand of sunblock and being in salt water all day with episodic drying of the salt water on my skin. On Saturday the diffuse pruritus (itching) persisted. Saturday evening in the tiny bathroom of our hotel room Stephanie noticed my urine was dark tea colored.

"What's that all about?" She asked.

"Liver's not working," I responded, trying desperately to sound poised and unfazed.

<This is bad, very bad. Try not to worry her.>

"It might be a side effect of one of the drugs," I said, looking away.

When I awoke the next morning I was yellow, including my eyes. In my reflection from the bathroom mirror I found myself staring at the return of the distended vein between my umbilicus (bellybutton) and the bottom of my breastbone. I was sick and going to get a lot sicker.

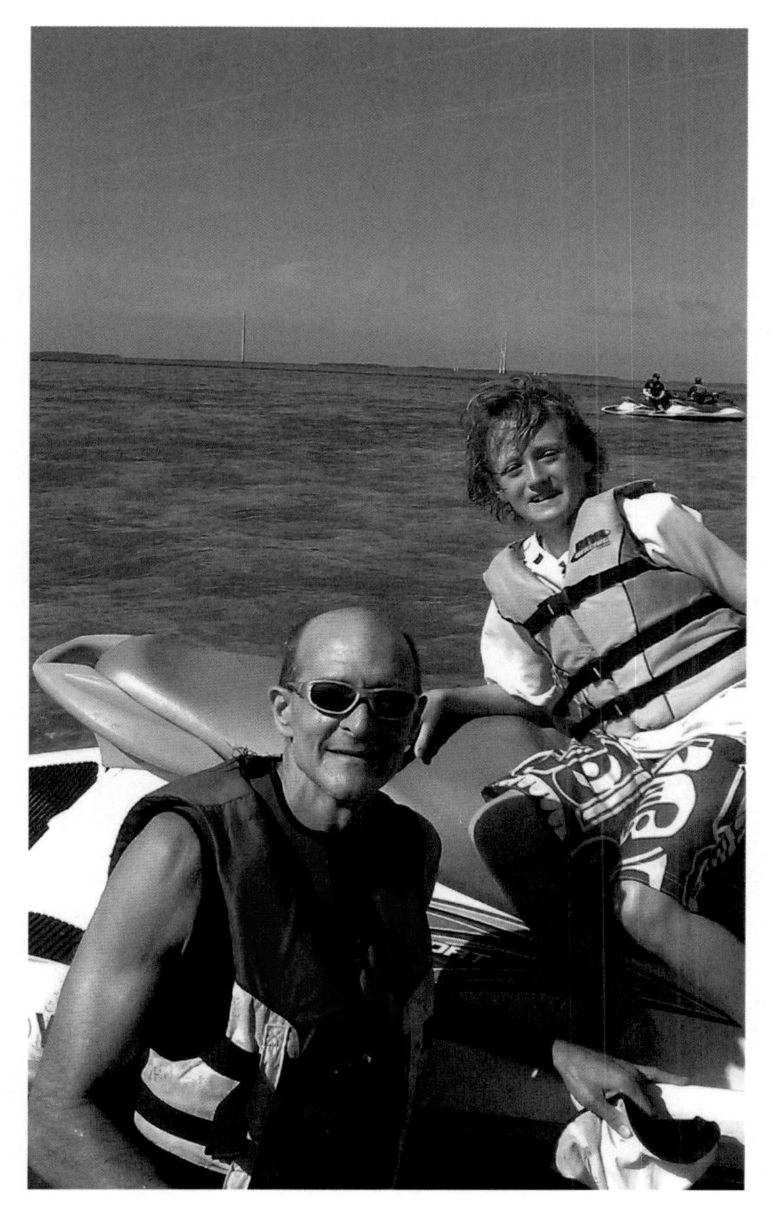

Figure 1
Jet Skiing around Key West with Nate

BEHIND YELLOW EYES
WITH APOLOGIES TO THE WHO

The final day of our vacation held no joy for me. We were scheduled to fly home the next day, so I focused on not subverting their fun. It was important that they not know my distress, at least not that day. No one commented on my new skin color and I didn't receive many questions so I concluded, correctly or not, I wasn't being a distraction. For the most part I stayed on the periphery of the group. Sunglasses and cover-ups helped hide the yellow.

Our trip home was easy and uneventful. Immediately after arriving home I called Dr. Roy Williams, my local oncologist, and described the situation. The conversation emphasized the urgency and the perilousness of my situation. Obviously I needed a CAT scan and a change in therapy, but what treatment and additional testing remained to be determined. I was to see him in his office the next day and we would start.

Dr. Williams inherited me as a patient when Dr. Alexander died. In fact Dr. Williams inherited all of Dr. Alexander's patients. As a physician and interested observer I tried to imagine what it was like for Dr. Williams when Dr. Alexander died. Dr. Alexander brought Dr. Williams into his solo practice some months earlier and was preparing Dr. Williams to be the principal partner in the next few years. Dr. Williams left work on Friday, August 26 as a "junior partner" and returned to work Monday, August 29 as the only physician for a busy oncology practice (more than 1000 patients I was told). The office staff had been with Dr. Alexander for many years and as an extended family they were grieving and in disbelief. Valiant was the word that best seemed to describe Dr. Williams' performance. Dr. Williams had seen me several times over the previous seven months, but not like this. You'll need to ask him his initial impression of me that day, if you are curious. I'm guessing it was something along the lines of 'This boy is gonna die!'

We began. CAT scan showed marked tumor progression in the liver with obstruction of the bile ducts[21]. The surgical consultant had nothing to offer. My bilirubin[22] was in double digits, normal being less than 1.5. Started a new chemo cocktail (capecitabine and temozolomide).

PinnacleHealth System's gastroenterologist wanted nothing to do with my situation and referred me to the Penn State Health Milton S. Hershey Medical Center (HMC) gastroenterologists for biliary stent[23] placement. Bilirubin continued to climb, liver was failing, lower extremities were swelling and weight was lost. Two weeks after return from Key West a biliary stent was placed at HMC. Bilirubin's climb continued. Liver failure worsened, swelling extended up to my buttocks severe enough that jeans couldn't pulled on. No longer yellow, my skin developed a greenish-gray hue. Desperate to buy time for the new chemo to work, if it was going to work, eight days after biliary stent placement direct biliary drains were placed through the wall of my torso into the liver. Large painful blisters formed on my hands. The blister fluid was yellow. Laying on the couch I felt my muscles dissolving, worst physical experience ever. Two days after drain placement, I saw Dr. Williams in his office. The next day he called me with lab results.

"Not good doc, bilirubin is up," he said.

"How high?" I asked.

"About 30," he replied.

<30>

In my thirty years of experience, albeit limited with respect to liver failure patients, every patient I ever saw with a bilirubin of 30 or greater died during that episode of liver failure, all of them!

---

[21] Bile ducts are tubular structures which convey bile from the liver to the small intestine.

[22] Bilirubin is a bile pigment formed from hemoglobin during the normal destruction of red blood cells. Small amounts are normally found circulating in the blood. Numerous pathologic conditions, particularly liver failure, result in increased amounts of bilirubin in the blood.

[23] A biliary stent is a slender artificial tube which is treaded into one of the larger bile ducts via the small intestine. It is sufficiently sturdy to prevent tumor from obstructing the bile duct into which it is placed.

"DARKNESS, DARKNESS"
THE YOUNGBLOODS

Although I had long expected this cancer to be the cause of my death, I was stunned by the speed with which this situation developed and by its finality. The certainty that I was actively in the dying process was profoundly unsettling.

In that moment no images of patients who had died in front of me, or whose last words were spoken to me came to mind. Faith permeates my life, but it did not come to mind. This was intensely personal. One of my touchstones came to mind: Time is Life, Life is Time. What to do with my precious, little remaining time?

Between keeping my head above water at work, living my life with my family and being a cancer patient, there was no residual time. I had spent as much time as possible with the kids and Nate would have an independent memory of me, but Maggie would not as she was less than three years old.

Over the years I had occasionally considered making a record of memories, thoughts, experiences, insights and recommendations in anticipation of questions they might ask of me, as they grew older. I had deliberated about the format, written or video and had a vague framework for the content. I could not manufacture the time required for the project; if only sleep wasn't essential. Consequently I had not made a record for parenting in absentia. Definitely the best use of my remaining time would be to make that record whether written, video or a combination; but which?

I was alone in the house. I wanted to talk with someone, but I didn't want the conversation to end with me in tears. That requirement determined who I could call. There was one relative with a no-nonsense attitude who had been very supportive, uplifting and in contact with me during the entire odyssey. I called him.

As we chatted I realized it was not possible for me to say "goodbye," to give voice to the fact that I would soon be dead. I mumbled something about it appeared that I did not have a lot of time left and I would keep him informed. I thanked him for his love and support over the years.

The conversation over, I resumed considering posterity. I decided on video recording myself and was preparing the specifics to record when my family arrived home. Time to be with them.

<I'll start tomorrow.>

A MOMENT OF TRANSCENDENCE

Occasionally we experience moments of transcendence. These moments are fleeting flashes of pure insight or recognition, which are not the product of thought, reasoning or our senses (sight, hearing, taste, smell and touch). However, such transcendence is transitory. Once experienced we want to experience more such moments, preferably on demand. The phenomena can frustrate and bewilder because the harder we try to force transcendence the farther we are from it. Worse yet, it is often only in retrospect that we recognize them. Our hearts must be open and our minds vigilant in order to receive and recognize these moments of transcendence when they occur.

[Thank you Kelly.]

It was the next morning and again I was alone in the house.

<I need to start on the archive for the kids… No, you don't… Yes, START NOW… No, it's not your time.>

In that instant, with absolute certainty I knew that I was not going to die at that time, despite all evidence and at least one expert opinion to the contrary[24]. I had transcended the here and now and knew the future. However, what did "not dying now" portend? I knew it meant more pain and suffering. It also meant a long road of recovery, but recovery to what level of function? A lower level of function certainly, but how much lower? On the positive side it meant my original goals remained, however unlikely, possible to reach. Seven years until Nate would be 18. Outliving dad might be the more difficult goal. Dad was 86 years old and chugging along. His goal was to live to be at least 97, the age at which his father and grandmother had died.

<Since I'm not going to die now I need a short-term goal.>

Establishing a short-term goal was quick and simple, get well enough to

---

[24] Dr. Williams later revealed that he did not expect me to survive until Easter.

play in the Hershey Country Club's Member-Guest Golf Tournament four months hence. The remainder was neither quick nor simple.

Cliché Alert

Hour by hour until the hours became days, day by day until the days became weeks I pulled, clawed, and dragged myself along Recovery Road. Walk up a flight of stairs without stopping, one minute walking on the elliptical trainer, walk down the driveway to get the mail and walk back up, lift a single plate, five repetitions each exercise, and so on. No attention was paid to diet while on Recovery Road. For eight years I had strictly avoided added and refined sugars and almost died anyway. So I consumed sweets whenever I wanted.

Although it would have been easy to focus on my frailty, lack of independence, the side-effects of the new chemo regimen or the glacial pace of improvement; the biliary drain was my primary torment for the next six weeks (Figure 1). About a week after placement I underwent a routine drain check in Interventional Radiology (IR). All seem to be in order and the drain flushed normally, so I was discharged to home. As Stephanie pulled the car into our garage I suddenly developed an intense shaking chill; almost certainly an indication that bacteria had entered my bloodstream (bacteremia) from the act of flushing the drain. It was back to my Emergency Department for a bucket of antibiotics and admission to the hospital. The next day, on antibiotics, I was discharged to home to rally from the setback. About two and half weeks later I returned to IR for a scheduled drain check. At that visit the biliary stent, which at no time had been helpful, was found to be clogged. The drain was revised slightly and was functioning normally. After the Interventional Radiologist exited the Radiology Techs were about to flush the drain in preparation for my discharge to home. I requested they not flush the drain because it would provide no useful information and I got bacteremic after the previous drain flush. The drain was flushed and I was moved to the post-procedure area to be discharged. I declined discharge explaining I would prefer to stay for 30-45 minutes in order to experience the shaking chills and fever in the post-procedure area rather than in my garage. On cue the shaking chill and fever occurred, but as we had seen the movie before it was antibiotics, observation then discharge to home; to rally from the setback.

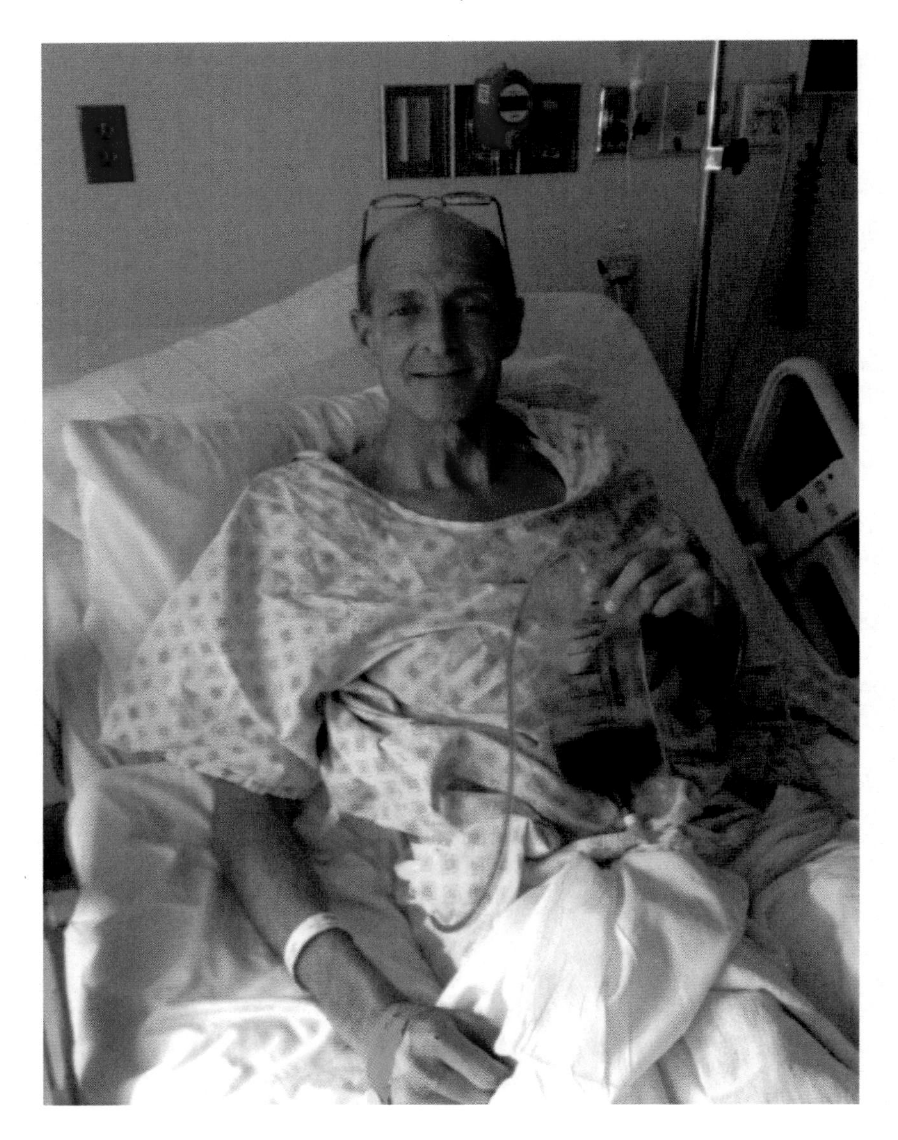

Figure 1
The lifesaving yet tormenting biliary drain

BUMPS IN THE ROAD
MAY, 2012

For various reasons we humans occasionally fixate on one small part of a big picture. So it was with me and my biliary drains. I resisted placement of the drains until it became clear they were the only remaining potentially life-saving treatment option available.

Now that I was starting to recover, I wanted them out! Their placement emphasized how gravely ill I was and as long as they were in they were a portal for infection. I wanted them out!

However they would not be removed until my bilirubin had declined to an acceptable level and the biliary stent in my liver had been removed. Far too slowly my bilirubin declined to an acceptable level and an appointment was made to have the stent removed.

The day for stent removal arrived. Fasted, hungry and uncaffeinated I waited with anticipation in the pre-procedure area of the gastroenterology suite at the Milton S. Hershey Medical Center (HMC).

I was moved into the procedure area. The gastroenterologist viewed the real-time x-ray (fluoroscopic) images of my abdomen and concluded the stent was no longer present. To his question, no I had not seen the stent pass in my stool. Nonetheless that is what must have occurred, as the stent was no longer visible in my liver. I was discharged home to schedule drain removal, which delighted me (Figure 1).

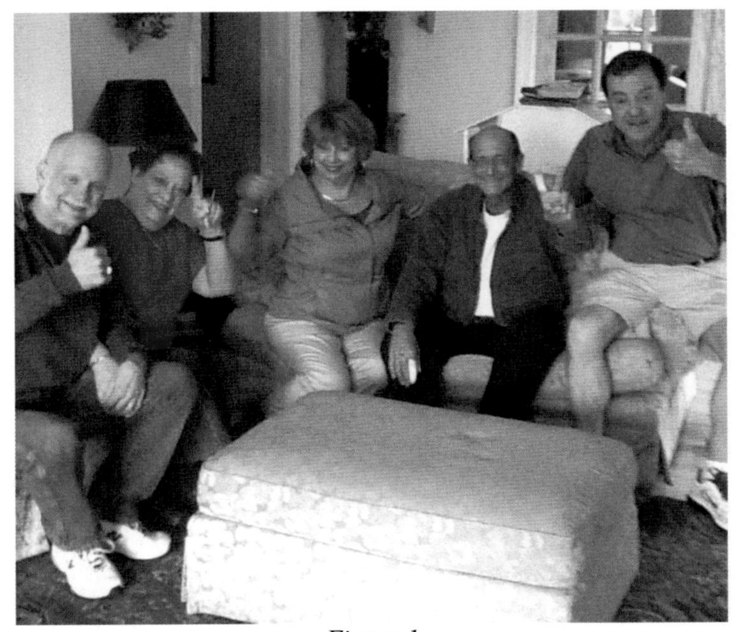

Figure 1
Anticipating drain removal with Cousins

The day for drain removal arrived! Fasted, hungry and uncaffeinated I waited on the procedure table for Jay, the interventional radiologist. Jay is a great doc and a good guy. As always I'm glad to see Jay, especially when he is smiling, which he was.

"Let's get those drains out," he said.

Now I was smiling. He fired up the fluoroscopy unit and positioned it over my abdomen.

"What did they tell you at Hershey?" he asked, no longer smiling.

"He said the stent was out, passed in the stool," I replied, also no longer smiling.

As Jay spun the viewing screen toward me my stomach sank, you know the feeling… impending, certain, major disappointment. Yes, there was a long biliary stent in my liver (Figure 2). No, the drain would not be removed today.

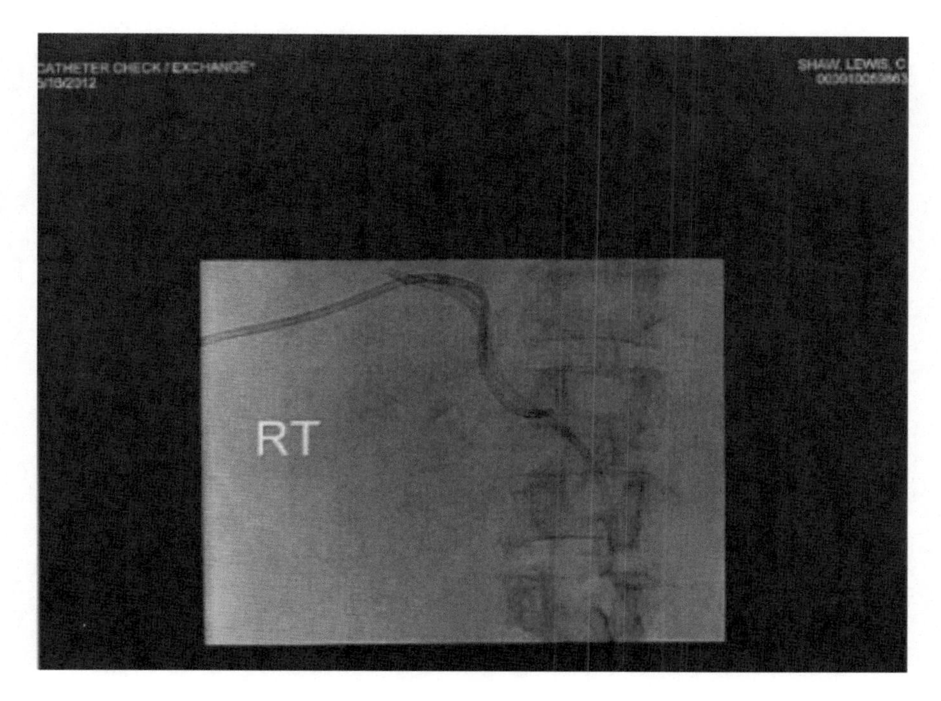

Figure 2

Another appointment was made to remove the stent. Fasted, hungry and uncaffeinated I waited in the pre-procedure area of the gastroenterology suite at the HMC. The gastroenterologist apologized, reviewed the images with me and it was into the procedure area to have the stent removed.

On May 24 the biliary drain was removed! It was replaced the following day. Removal of the drain was fast and painless. After removal an ultrasound showed no free fluid in my abdomen indicating no bile was leaking into the abdominal cavity from the liver.

Important information because bile leaking into the abdominal cavity causes an intensely painful inflammatory condition called bile peritonitis. Still not permitted to drive, Stephanie chauffeured me home where she left me to eat while she got on with her day. Oddly I did not feel hungry. About half an hour later the pain started. About half an hour later I was on the phone to Steph.

"Sorry to interrupt, but you need to come home and take me back to the hospital," I said.

"Why?" she asked.

"I'm having a lot of pain."

"Okay."

"As soon as you can, please."

About half an hour later Steph arrived home to find me pale and sweaty. I did not want to move or take a deep breath. Slowly I shuffled to the garage. I was dreading the ride to the hospital, as I knew each bump in the road would be excruciatingly painful. About half an hour later I was sitting on a bench outside my Emergency Department (ED) retching, having been unable to walk from the car to the door of the ED.

<This is embarrassing and very uncool.>

In a wheelchair I was transported into my own ED, where I drew a crowd. Even when metastatic cancer doesn't kill it certainly humiliates.

<I hate this, I hate this, I hate this!>

The staff were having difficulty starting an intravenous line and getting the cardiac monitor patches to stick because I was sweating profusely and needed to sit upright.

"I'm sorry to be difficult," I apologized, "but I can't lay flat, the pain is too intolerable supine.
Bile peritonitis," I continued, self-diagnosing, "My biliary drain was pulled a couple of hours ago."

My return to the Radiology suite was expedited. The radiology techs attempted to get me into the CT scanner.

"I KNOW I need to be supine for the scan, but I can't get into that position because the pain is too great," I pleaded.

"We can't give you any pain medication until the Radiologist is here," the tech countered.

My vulgar response was prevented by the arrival of the interventional radiologist.

"After you've signed the consent for the paracentesis[25], we can give you pain medication." He began, following the ritual which I've long thought is coercive, but which had necessarily evolved during the decades before my training in response to liability concerns about patient competence to consent to or decline recommended treatment after receiving narcotics. I signed the consent before he could review the potential complications or ask if I had questions.

From the radiology suite I ricocheted off the ED to an inpatient room. Still in severe pain I was provided with a patient controlled analgesia (PCA) pump[26] for pain control. I have a healthy respect for narcotic analgesics so I pushed the button enough to subdue the pain to a level where I was less sweaty and could tolerate the pain of breathing.

Stephanie had been with me the entire afternoon and I felt better with her there. However it was getting toward evening and the kids needed her at home. We were discussing the next day and she was preparing to leave when an unexpected visitor arrived. Janice, the Director of the Pharmacy Department was one of the most intelligent, determined, hardest working people at Pinnacle. I suspect 70 hours was a short work week for her. Janice was a friend and had been a highly valued colleague with whom I worked for more than 15 years. She looked at me and asked how often I was pushing the PCA button. After I responded, she checked the pump settings.

"Give me that," she said, grabbing the button from me.

Push, push, push…

---

[25] Paracentesis is the passage of a needle and catheter through the abdominal wall into the abdominal cavity with the subsequent removal of fluid, in this case bile.

[26] A PCA (Patient Controlled Analgesia) pump is a device used for pain control via the intravenous infusion of a narcotic analgesic, such as morphine, Dilaudid or fentanyl. The device includes a pump which infuses the narcotic at a pre-set basal rate and a mechanism for the patient to self-administer additional narcotic if the pain is not controlled by the continuous infusion. A maximum dosing limit is predetermined and the device settings are programed to prevent administration of narcotic in excess of the limit.

"That will be better," she said looking at Stephanie reassuringly.

<Do they have an insurance policy on me I don't know about?>

Sure enough I did feel better, a lot better. The pain didn't seem much diminished, but I no longer cared about it. I stopped sweating and was able to breathe satisfactorily. I was going to be able to sleep.

[Thank you Janice!]

Back in Radiology the next day a drain was replaced through the wall of my torso into the abdominal cavity to drain the leaking bile. Despite the circumstances I was optimistic, thinking the surface of the liver would heal rapidly stopping the bile leak so the drain could be removed in several days, not several weeks. One week later, on June 1, 2012 the drain was removed. I couldn't take a deep breath because of pain, exercise, lift more than 5 pounds, get in a swimming pool or swing a golf club; but I was finally free of the drains. However, it appeared I had established a goal beyond my reach, as it was less than nine weeks until the Member-Guest Tournament.

Epilogue

The HMC patient representative was very pleasant on the phone, as is typical for patient representatives. I explained the sequence of events, which necessitated a second trip to the Gastroenterology procedure suite and emphasized I was not interested in a quality assurance review, disciplinary or legal action at this juncture, but I wanted to be certain that only one of the visits was billed.

"But you did need to have the stent removed, correct?" she said, attempting to get me to concede the point.

"Yes, but only once," I replied sternly. "So you can choose the visit to bill, but only one okay?"

"Yes, I see," she replied.

"STRENGTH"
THE ALARM
JUNE 2012

Inspiration sometimes arrives unexpectedly.

The Solstice Cup was a small local youth soccer tournament, which a neighboring soccer club was holding as a fundraiser. As best I could determine, none of us wanted to be in the tournament. The coaches said they didn't want to enter the team, but felt obliged to as a favor to the tournament organizers. The players, all 11 years old, seemed uninterested. The boys were interested in summer vacation from school, family vacations and the pool, but not team soccer. We parents, after a long winter-spring season, were looking forward to the two-month hiatus before the resumption of practice for the fall season, not another tournament. For a while it appeared there wouldn't be enough players in town to enter the team. The apathy was not restricted to our team as one of the other entered teams reportedly withdrew shortly before the tournament kickoff because of an insufficient number of players. Me? I was elated to be alive and tolerating the chemotherapy. I was recovering slowly. Still quite weak I fatigued easily and had very sensitive, fragile skin, among many other annoying signs and symptoms.

However, it ultimately came to pass that the Hershey Demolition boys U12 soccer team played in the 2012 Solstice Cup Tournament, a two day eight versus eight event. The previously mentioned withdrawal of a team left only four teams in the Demolition's age group, which resulted in a bizarre format. Day one was round robin play plus one additional game. The results of the day one games were used to seed the teams for day two which was double elimination play, all teams starting day two with clean records. The four games on day one resulted in 80 minutes of aggregate game time for each team. On day two all of the games had 20 minute halves. The Demolition would have nine players and both coaches on day one, but only eight players (no substitutes) and one coach on day two.

Day one of the tournament was played under cloudless, brilliant blue skies. The air was still, the temperature in the low 80s and humidity was low. The Demolition won all of their day one matches convincingly. As the coaches summarized with the players, we parents concocted our plans for day two. Among the parents was my 86-year-old father. It was almost one year to the day since he buried his wife of 60 years, but he would not miss this for it was his world. Given the circumstances, our parental plan was logical and efficient. At the conclusion of the next day's 8 a.m. match we would all go out for breakfast, return home for the boys to relax and maybe go to the pool for a short while. We would return in the afternoon for the championship match.

Except for a few afternoon clouds the day one weather was cloned for day two. First up for the boys was the team from Lititz, which they easily defeated on day one. A very famous person once wrote about *The best-laid schemes...* Our parental scheme lasted for less than 20 minutes. By halftime it was clear the Demolition was destined for the losers' bracket as Lititz completely dominated the match from the opening kickoff. We parents scrambled. There would be no time for breakfast as there were only 20 minutes between matches. Some parents went for snacks, drinks and ice while others set up the canopy, chairs and coolers. There was an unspoken silver lining for me, a second loss would end the soccer day early permitting more time at the pool and I could get out of the sun.

The second loss did not come in either of the next two matches, as the boys earned narrow victories in each of the two. Coach Scott rested the players by rotating each through the goalie position. Between matches they possessed the shade of the canopy. With 120 minutes of soccer behind them the Demolition exited the losers' bracket to face the rested Lititz team. In order to win the tournament the Demolition needed to beat Lititz twice, a loss in either match and the Demolition would be runner-up. The fresh legs of the Lititz team were apparent as they breezed to a two-goal lead in the first half. I was feeling weak, lightheaded, dizzy and more than a little selfish.

<Just as well they lose this one before I faint, that would embarrass my son and worry my dad. Dad, I should check on him.>

I walked the few meters along the sideline to where dad was sitting.

"How are you holding up?" I asked.

"It's not over yet," he replied, not looking at me.

Hoping he would provide an excuse for leaving I persisted.

"How are you feeling?"

"I'm fine," he emphasized, still focused on the field.

<Shit>

"I'm going to get a water. Do you want one?"

"I'll get one at the half."

Halftime came and went. The Demolition scored to get within one goal, but were unable to get the equalizer and time had almost run out. They worked hard to the end and didn't quit I thought, feeling fatigued, weaker, more lightheaded; but not quite so selfish. Then bang-bang-bang the ball was behind their goalie rolling into the middle of the goal, with one of our forwards, also behind their goalie to shield the ball. No off-sides. Nothing to prevent the goal, except the goalie?! The Lititz goalie pulled our forward down from behind, dove over the falling forward and got one hand on the ball at the goal line-no goal! The play was impressively athletic and impressively illegal, but would the penalty be called? There was only one official per match for this tournament and this ref hadn't called much against either side. He hesitated… some yelling from all around… still nothing… I heard Coach Scott's voice… the penalty was called. A penalty kick (PK) was awarded to the Demolition and the Lititz goalie was given a red card, out for the remainder of that game. The penalty kick was made, tying the score at the end of regulation time. By tournament format this match would be decided by penalty kicks, not overtime. The score was tied at four after five rounds of PKs. The next team to miss, and opponent make, loses the match. Make… Make… Miss… Make… Demolition win! A 20 minute break before the final match, in which the starting Lititz goalie was eligible to play. During the break we congregated at the canopy. One of parents asked Coach Scott if the boys were complaining.

"No, not a word," he said "It brings a tear to the eye."

Lititz again started strong and took the lead. Now at almost every stoppage of play one or two substitutes came on the field for Lititz. Watching the substitutions the Demolition players Alex, Anthony,

Brady, Colby, Chris, Evan, Luke and Nate simply stood where they were waiting for play to resume. We became increasingly worried about the heat stress on our boys and during one of the stoppages a dad cracked, taking a water bottle to his son on the field. The player grudgingly took the bottle from his dad, poured some water over his head and tossed the bottle at his retreating father. When the tying goal came I was standing next to Alex's grandmother.

"I'm getting chills watching them play," she said, her voice cracking with emotion.

<ENOUGH! Enough focusing on yourself. After 180 minutes of soccer without substitution the players aren't complaining. Dad is not complaining. Their coach, an orthopedic surgeon and former professional athlete, is moved by their performance and a strong grandmother is getting choked up. Cancer, chemotherapy you are not stronger than me today, not today! So f**k you cancer, f**k you!>

With 10 minutes remaining in the match the Demolition scored the go-ahead goal. As the cheering subsided I said, to no one in particular, that the next 10 minutes would seem very long. Five minutes later Alex's grandmother said that it seemed like time was standing still. Lititz scored the equalizer and was looking strong on the attack again. Less than one minute remained when, against the flow of play one of our forwards broke loose up the middle with the ball. He was taken down by a hard tackle well outside the penalty area, but a foul was called and a direct kick was awarded. The goalie set his defense and the kick was taken. As the ball sailed over the defensive wall everybody moved; the players in the wall jumped, all the players not in the wall raced toward the goal and the goalie moved to make a play on the ball.

In my mind's eye the ball is still hanging there in the air. Of course it isn't. It hit the crossbar bouncing straight down into the field of play where it was instantly volleyed into the back of the net by Anthony. Goal Demolition! The goal was immediately followed by an intense, very dangerous final attack by Lititz. Pinball around the Demolition goal. The ball came to the foot of a Demolition defender, Alex who turned and kicked the ball as far out of bounds as he could. Final whistle, game over, tournament over. Demolition win! Pure joy! The players jumped into a pile on the field.

After the awards ceremony with obligatory pictures (Figure 1) we loaded our vehicles to depart.

"Let me carry that," said my friend Greg, seeing that I was struggling with the canopy.

"I sincerely appreciate the offer Greg, but if I don't do these these things myself, I won't regain any strength."

Epilogue

After driving Dad home and seeing he was settled back in his air-conditioned house, I made my way to the pool. As I walked to where the other parents were sitting, food was being brought to the tables. I hadn't seen the boys in the pool as I walked by, so asked where they were. My attention was directed to the grass area where they were... playing soccer.

[Thank you Scott for your considerable time and effort over the years for the boys. More than your countless hours, thank you for being an outstanding role model.]

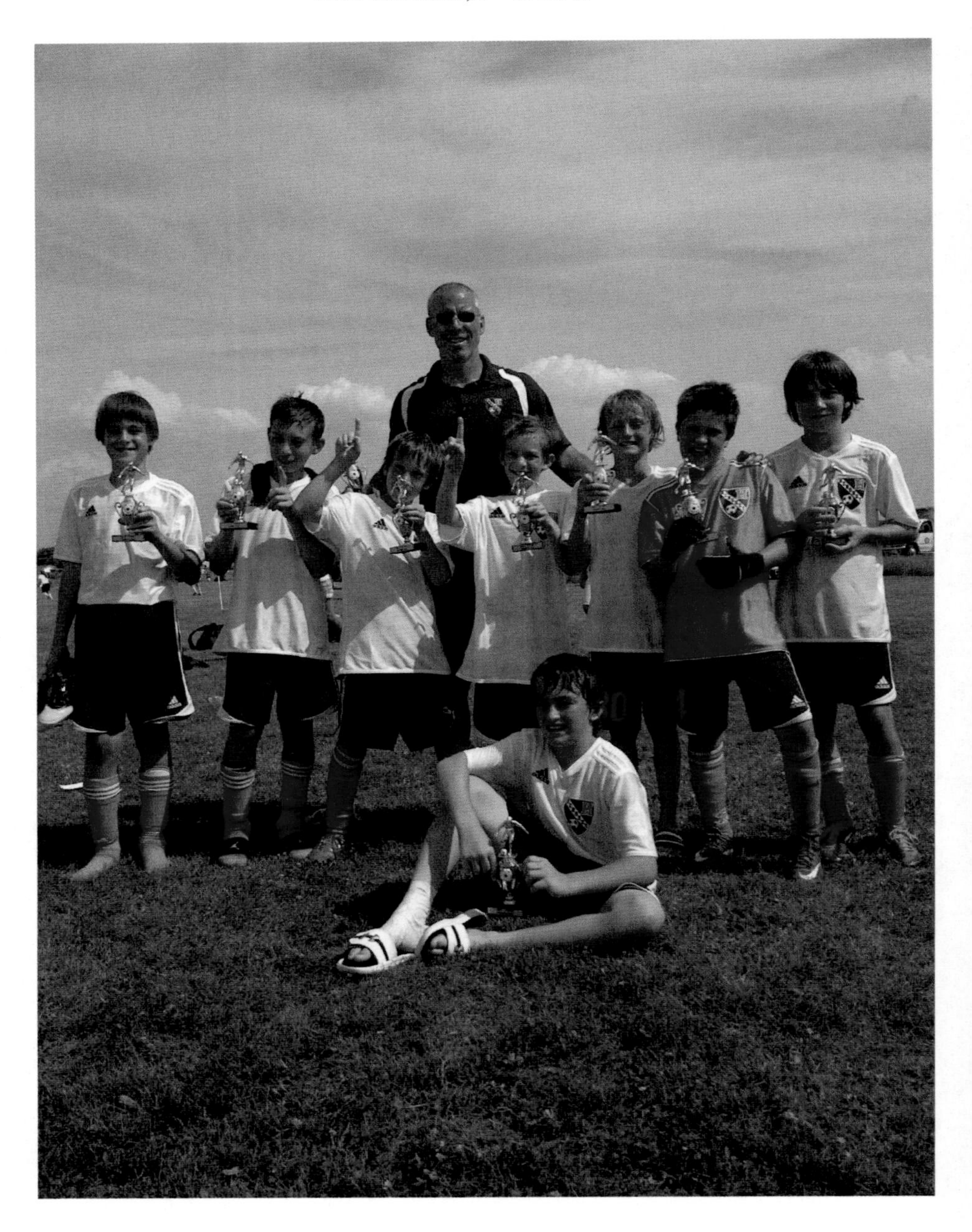

Figure 1
The Hershey Demolition – 2012 Solstice Cup Champions

A TEA PARTY

I regained enough strength to play in the Member-Guest Golf Tournament at the Hershey Country Club. I maintain we were soundly defeated not because I was hitting the ball three clubs shorter than before my near-death episode, or because playing nine holes of golf from a cart was exhausting to the point of not being able to take a practice swing by the end of each match, or because I didn't practice the week before the tournament, but because my partner prepared for the tournament by going on a family vacation instead of practicing. While I had reached my goal of playing in the Member-Guest, my assumption that I would return to work proved false.

Clearly I was not going to recover the physical and mental capabilities to perform my job. Additionally working in a hospital with my level of immunocompromise would jeopardize my life. Finally it was apparent the intensity of the unremitting job stress was a significant contributor to the near fatal episode of disease progression. Disregard my slow, grudging acceptance of the situation, Dr. Williams was not going to permit me to return to work, saving my life a second time.

[Thanks Doc!]

The emotional pain associated with broadcasting my resignation was severe. Progressing beyond a normal grief reaction, I became depressed. Despite my healthy family, despite surviving a near fatal episode of disease progression, despite all my blessings I was very depressed.

The PinnacleHealth System had a tradition of celebrating the retirement of those individuals who had served the System for many years with a Retirement Tea. The Teas were festive, memorable events and not an everyday occurrence. They wanted to honor me with a Tea and emotionally I was deeply moved. When my colleague, Christian, called with the invitation I was hesitant because I was depressed and thought the event might be emotionally overwhelming. Christian emphasized that many people wanted an opportunity to say "goodbye" to me. As I considered the invitation I realized there were many people I wanted to thank and would otherwise not have an opportunity to do so. I accepted the invitation and the date was set for November 8, 2012. As the date for the Tea approached my feelings of depression subsided. Slow improvement of the cancer continued. When the day of the Tea arrived I was joyful. The event was festive and I was overwhelmed, with gratitude. I will always cherish the memories of the event (Figure 1).

One of the best days ever.

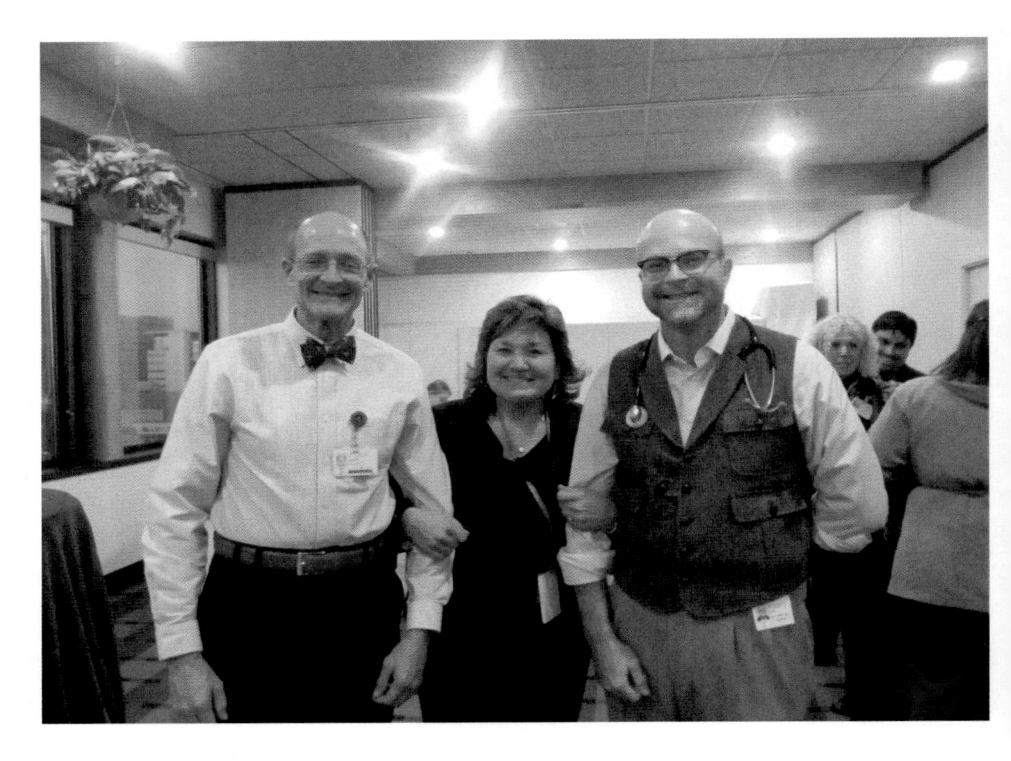

Figure 1
At a Tea Party with Two Lifesavers
Janice Dunsavage, Director of Pharmacy and Dr. Roy Williams

ASKING AN UNEXPECTED QUESTION

As Chair of the Pharmacy and Therapeutics Committee I was an ex officio member of its subcommittees, including the Oncology Subcommittee. This particular meeting of the Oncology Subcommittee had yet to start and I was chatting with one of the oncology nurses, Amy. Amy is an exceptionally good nurse and has an appealing sense of humor. She and her colleagues provided the life-sustaining care, which I had received in the outpatient infusion center during the previous year.

<Maybe an opportunity to have a little fun.>

"What did you think when you first met me?" I asked Amy.

Amy responded immediately, "I remember my first impression of you – 'Oh my, this boy is yellow!' - You were a color that is difficult to describe, unless you've seen it."

"Did you think I was going to die?"

She hesitated.

"Come on you can say, it's been a year."

"I wasn't sure."

[Profound thanks to the 2012-13 staff of the PinnacleHealth Hospitals Medical Outpatient Unit.]

TEN YEARS AFTER
MARCH 3, 2014

Unless otherwise obliged I spend little time recognizing event anniversaries, fundamentally because my Time's Arrow flies so swiftly to and through them. The dates of life-changing events embed themselves in one's mind in a manner, which obliges recognition. However, even those dates tend to sneak up on me.

The day I received the diagnosis of incurable metastatic neuroendocrine cancer, March 3 obliges my recognition. The emotion associated with the anniversary has evolved over the years without any conscious action on my part.

As the years became a decade the anniversary rage metamorphosed into anniversary triumph. As the anniversary of my diagnosis isn't precisely personal for anyone else and given my baseline attitude toward event anniversaries, I hadn't planned anything special for March 3, 2014. So I sent some emails.

To family and friends

"Ten years ago today I received the diagnosis of incurable, metastatic neuroendocrine cancer. The decade is a testament to the power of faith, prayer, love and hate (Oh yes, I HATE this disease!).

Profound thanks and appreciation for your love, prayers, support and assistance. I look forward to sending a similar communiqué ten years from today.

With much love to you all."

To Dr. Steve

"I replayed the episode a few times over the years and there is no one who could have delivered the news in the manner which you did. You are the consummate professional and have been a great role model over the years. It is unfortunate that more young physicians did not have the opportunity to work with you.

I was very fortunate to have you as a physician and continue to be even more fortunate to have you as a friend. I'll plan something a bit more formal to celebrate the 20th anniversary. Maybe I'll even have a drink, probably not.

Best to you… "

To cousin Mira

"One of the most profound moments of this entire odyssey was during our early phone conversation when you made the unsolicited offer to donate part of your liver to me. That was the most touching, heartfelt, unexpected act of love and generosity which I've ever received. I will always cherish that memory (However, I'm really, really glad the offer did not need to be accepted!).

Please let me know if there's anything I can ever do for you.

I'm planning to host an organized celebration for the 20th anniversary, so please 'save the date'!

Hope all is well with you."

To Pastor Kelly

"One of the most under emphasized lessons of The Cross is that 'suffering is required.' Suffering tests the individual's heart, soul and faith. It's easy to be a good person and a good Christian during the cakewalk parts of life, so it is under adversity that we are tested. I'm just trying to pass the test.

As always I'm glad to do what I can to help anyone you know in a similar position.

Best to you and your loved ones."

<Wow, it has been 10 years. What about the next 10 years?... You know that is one aspect of the future, which is not possible to predict, except that you will suffer... True, so continue to give maximum daily effort and pray for the best, but prepare for the worst... Yep.>

Without treatment my disease was stable for about two years (spring 2013 - spring 2015). During that interval my constant supplement regimen was:

AHCC (Active Hexose Correlated Compound) 750 mg daily
CoQ 10 – 100mg daily
Cranberry concentrate 500mg twice a day
Essiac 2 oz. twice a day
Fish oil 1g daily
Flax oil 1g daily
Ginseng (Panax) 100mg daily
Greens 1 scoop daily
Milk Thistle 250mg twice a day
Multivitamin w/ minerals (no Iron) one daily
N-Acetyl Cysteine 500mg twice a day
Probiotics daily in evening
Raspberry powder ½ Tbsp. daily
Vitamin C (ester) 500mg daily
Vitamin D (3) 1000 IU daily (not taken during the summer months)

DECISION-MAKING AND INTEGRATING TREATMENTS

Most patients with active metastatic cancer use some type of self-selected alternative, complementary, nontraditional and/or integrative treatment, most commonly oral supplements. It is important to convey clearly my definitions of certain terms so my support of integrating treatments won't be misinterpreted.

Alternative: Treatment which differs in scope and approach from traditional science-based treatments. Acupuncture, acupressure, aromatherapy, homeopathy, therapeutic touch, ozone, fasts, bowel cleansing, hydrotherapy, music therapy and reflexology are examples of treatments, which are often considered alternative.

Complementary: Nontraditional treatment added to traditional science-based treatment, often with the intent of maximizing the therapeutic effect of or ameliorating the side-effects of the traditional treatment. Examples include oral ginger to alleviate nausea and ginseng for fatigue.

Integrative: Treatment, which combines traditional and alternative treatments.

Traditional: Treatment based on conventional medical education and scientific evidence.

Proven: Surprisingly difficult to define because there are no uniform, generally accepted criteria for establishing proof. Phrases such as "a reasonable degree of medical certainty" or "a preponderance of evidence" might be satisfactory for legal purposes, but they do not necessarily meet the scientific burden of proof. The level of proof required to prove something is highly variable depending upon who is certifying/asserting that the thing/concept is proven and the relevance of the proof to the individual. If randomized, double-blind, placebo-controlled studies are required for proof then it remains unproven that parachutes are beneficial when jumping from a flying aircraft. Not only is "proven" elusive, but occasionally it is also unimportant or irrelevant such as when one is enrolling in an experimental trial, which by its nature is seeking to obtain proof. Despite the entanglements, when deciding to undergo treatment "proven" or "not proven" is more important than the monikers alternative, complementary or traditional.

While a detailed analysis or discussion of treatments is beyond the scope of this book, there are fundamental analytical problem-solving principles to assist in making your treatment decisions.

First, do no harm. The founding principle of all healthcare. It is much easier written than accomplished as all treatments have the potential for harm. The harm can be forgoing treatment, which will work/be effective for treatment which won't (Steve Jobs). Very often it is underestimating, overlooking or dismissing the potential for harm. The term "risk-benefit" can increase the underappreciation of harm because the term implies benefit is associated with the treatment while there is only the risk of harm. Few treatments are guaranteed to benefit. Your decision-making is better served by analyzing a treatment in terms of the potential for harm and the potential for benefit. This analysis must be performed in the context of your distinct personal situation. Probiotics, for example, are beneficial in a number of situations and important in some. However systemic infections have been caused by some probiotics supplements and the potential for harm is such that the probiotic yeast Saccharomyces boulardii is contraindicated in immunocompromised patients.

The lure of physiologic plausibility: A single physiologic process or biochemical pathway is isolated and a treatment is demonstrated to have a beneficial effect on the isolated process or pathway. Consequently it is physiologically plausible for the treatment to benefit the patient. Since no physiologic process or biochemical pathway proceeds in isolation in humans, it is not surprising when the treatment is found to be ineffective, or even harmful in patients. The medical literature is replete with instances of physiologically plausible treatments failing to benefit patients. The power of physiologic plausibility, especially when coupled with the profit motive, is such that multiple studies with negative results sometimes are insufficient to prevent further attempts to prove benefit. The persistence of a physiologically plausible treatment despite negative experimental results in humans is aided by the fact that it is difficult to prove a negative. Determined, resourceful proponents of the treatment can argue the timing, dose, duration and sometimes route of treatment were incorrect and responsible for the negative results.

Pigs don't equal people. Although some people are pigs, for analytic experimental purposes only humans equal people. Experimentally determining something is effective in nonhuman animals does not promise the same results in humans. Near the end of 2005 I began taking a colostrum oral supplement to support my immune system, based on preliminary reports of animal research. Within two months of starting colostrum my platelet count[27] began to decline, which I attributed to the Sutent I was taking as low platelet counts are a common side effect of that drug. Over approximately the next two months my platelet count neared a dangerously low level which would have necessitated a reduction in the Sutent dose or stopping the drug. About the same time I discovered a brief report which implied a possible association between colostrum supplementation and low platelet counts. I immediately discontinued the colostrum with prompt acceptable improvement of my platelet count.

What is the denominator? Purveyors of alternative treatments often proclaim an instance of the treatment under discussion being successful. However all details of the case history are not provided and we don't know the denominator, how many patients underwent the treatment without benefit. If the promoted treatment is effective, is it effective in 1 in 100 or 1 in 100 million patients? A friend and former colleague of mine underwent intravenous vitamin C therapy for metastatic esophageal cancer… and died.

Beware of epidemiology and hearsay. Epidemiology is the study of the determinants, dynamics and distribution of diseases or health related events in specified populations. Epidemiology has very important administrative, research and insurance uses and is essential in the formulation and implementation of public health policy. The importance of population statistics is undeniable, they quantify the likelihood of something occurring or not occurring in a population. However they cannot foretell if that something will or will not occur in the individual. I have never investigated, read or inquired about the survival statistics of my disease, because those statistics don't apply to me the individual and they might be anxiety provoking. Hearsay evidence or reports also do not foretell what will occur in the individual. Statements such as "I was told…", "What I have heard from friends is…" and the like are not

[27] Platelets are irregularly shaped cell fragments found circulating in the blood. They are an essential component of normal blood clotting.

helpful. Metastatic cancer is an absurdly complex disease and each one of us is unique and unimaginably complex. Consequently one's response to a treatment and the side-effects experienced are individual. If you decide to undergo a treatment your response to treatment and the side-effects you experience will be yours and no one else's.

When faced with a complicated decision about treatment keep the following running in the background of your thinking:
If what you are doing is working, favor its continuation;
If what you are doing is not working, change what you're doing;
If you absolutely don't know what to do, don't make changes and get more information. Information and a bit of time often clarify the next step;
If the alternative is disease progression, stable disease is satisfactory. If your disease is bedrock stable then the treatment is helping; probably not as much as you want it to help, but it is helping.

When I was diagnosed the pressure I felt to be cured of the incurable was intense, at times almost overwhelming. Ongoing pressure, internal and external to undergo treatment is an obligatory part of having the disease.

THAT WHICH IS TRUE

Most of what follows is not original and includes aphorisms that have been told and retold, written and rewritten since humans first conceived them. However they are vital, critically important and warrant inclusion.

The first group is related to the disease, the second collection are the axioms of earthly life. Never overlook, minimize, dismiss or forget them. Always have them running in the background when you are thinking.

<u>Embrace your faith.</u> Unless you believe your faith advocates harming others, in which case - drop dead, please.

<u>Live your life.</u> Make every effort not to define yourself as your disease.

<u>Know your disease.</u> Become informed. Of paramount importance is establishing the urgency of your situation; how aggressive and how widespread is the disease? Not everyone gets cured, there is no equality of outcome.

<u>Cancer never sleeps and neither should you.</u> Commit to staying informed. Learn from your experiences and those of others. Be active in your treatment. Metaphor aside, sleep is essential. Getting the proper amount of good quality sleep is vital. Consequently, to the extent possible, you must minimize all factors which interfere with your sleep.

<u>Obtain multiple medical opinions.</u> Repeat as needed, such as when the situation changes significantly.

<u>The treatment should not be worse than the disease.</u> It's easy to kill cancer. What is hard is not killing the patient. Stable disease is often satisfactory and satisfactory is underrated.

<u>Don't overlook prevention and routine maintenance in/of any other body system.</u> Understand the human organism is completely, totally integrated. All body systems are elegantly interconnected and mutually

dependent.

Having goals is essential. Maintain focus on your goals. One simple goal for those of us with incurable disease is to stay alive long enough for some brilliant people to develop treatment which results in the long term absence of detectable disease.

The only absolute contraindication to exercise is fever. If you find yourself in a funk – MOVE!

Seek that which is uplifting. Genuine laughter corresponds to an absence of fear.

Don't give up, but know when to quit.

The Fifteen Axioms

[I never did get around to making a video archive for the kids, so your forbearance is politely requested.]

1 Earthly life is unfair.

2 No one can change Axiom One.

3 Any time spent in anguish of Axioms One and Two is wasted time.

4 It's always about time (and timing).

5 Nature is indifferent, change is inevitable.

6 The price of perfection is infinite.

7 The individual chooses the meaning to give her/his life.

8 To avoid criticism say nothing, do nothing, be nothing.

9 Nothing of significance is easy to accomplish.

10 Never surrender to fear.

11 Never give up, but know when to quit.

12 Recognize dangerous/crazy people and avoid them.

13 It is not possible to reason with a sick mind. This includes intoxicated brains and zealots, all of whom mistake their psychopathology for enlightenment.

14 Bad information is worse than no information.

15 Don't panic!

One of the most powerful yet overlooked attributes of the mind is its ability to choose its attitude. Each and every day you get to choose your attitude toward life. Choose strength and good luck!

APPENDICES

Fox Chase Cancer Center IRB# 07-033 Current IRB Approval: 07/10/2007
Page 10 of 17

Will your medical information be kept private?
We will do our best to make sure that the personal information in your medical record will be kept private. However, we cannot guarantee total privacy. Your personal information may be given out if required by law. If information from this study is published or presented at scientific meetings, your name and other personal information will not be used.

Organizations that may look at and/or copy your medical records for research, quality assurance, and data analysis include:

- The Food and Drug Administration (FDA)
- Governmental agencies in other countries where the drug may be considered for approval
- Fox Chase Cancer Center
- Novartis Pharmaceuticals Corporation and its authorized agents

You will be given a separate form to review regarding the steps we will take to guard your privacy as part of your taking part in the research study. By signing that additional authorization, you will be providing your consent for use and disclosure described in that form connected with your taking part in this research study.

What are the costs?
Some procedures such as x-rays and lab tests may not be covered by insurance. This means you may have to pay for them. You need to check with your insurance company to find out what will be paid for by insurance if you take part in a research study. We will discuss possible costs with you before the research study begins

You will receive the study drug RAD001 free of charge.

If your insurance will not pay for medicines you may need to help with side effects, you may have to pay for them.

Will you be compensated?
You will not get paid for taking part in this research study.

If you are harmed because of the research study, we will provide the medical care to treat that harm. However, you may have to pay for this treatment. Fox Chase Cancer Center has not set aside funds to pay your salary if you cannot work or for any other damages if you are harmed because of the research study.

If the study was done correctly and you are hurt by the study drug, Novartis will pay for all reasonable medical bills that your insurance company does not pay. These are the only bills that Novartis will pay. If the Study Site or someone who works for them caused your harm, Novartis will not pay your medical bills. If you are hurt because you did not follow instructions, Novartis will not pay your medical bills. If your disease or the treatment of your disease caused your harm, Novartis will not pay your medical bills.

Appendix A
How does that happen?

NEUROPHILOSOPHY [$ the 3 bowl exp]

• Classic Pulvolist
Empiricist
or Existentialist

└ father Pulvols
- date of inception 4.14.80

** Neural adapt. - Δ in resp. (usually ↓) in resp to ⊕
- not the same a psychosensory adapt.

Type 1 ↔ w/ Merkle cell

Type 2 ↔ w/ Ruffinian receptor

unit recept. field - receptive field of 1 neuron

[unit ⟺ neuron]

Gradation of stim (1) rel. weak stim (@ or near threshold) - not all receptors on same area have same threshold

slowly adapting
rapidly adapting
C. 1.
total thresholds
intensity of ⊕ →

(2) frequency code - operates @ levels > thresh.;
coding of stim. w/ the rate firing

C. 2.
log # of # spikes
log ⊕ →

- the code for ⊕ occurs @ the level of the generator potential !!

C. 3.
spikes / sec
generator potent. →

Appendix B
"Neurophilosophy" coined?

Made in the USA
Middletown, DE
06 June 2019